Common Sense Pediatrics

Combining Alternative and Traditional Medicine in Everyday Practice

by

S. Cornelia Franz MD

AuthorHouse™
1663 Liberty Drive, Suite 200
Bloomington, IN 47403
www.authorhouse.com
Phone: 1-800-839-8640

First published by AuthorHouse   11/22/2008

ISBN: 978-1-4343-6910-9 (sc)

Library of Congress Control Number: 2008910162

Printed in the United States of America
Bloomington, Indiana

This book is printed on acid-free paper.

Dedication

This book is dedicated to Joe, Daniel, and Patrick.
I love you and thank you for all you have taught me.
Without you, this book would not be possible.

Contents

Chapter One

Finding the Physician/Practice that fits your Needs

Choosing a physician for yourself or your child is an important decision. I am often asked what questions someone should ask, and how to choose. Common sense will answer most of the questions you have.

Statistically, most people start looking for a physician who is geographically close to their home. I highly encourage patients not to let *convenience* be their guide. Next, most patients look to see if the physician they are thinking about is on their insurance plan. While that can be important, paying out of pocket may in the long run be a less expensive venture.

The best resource for finding a physician you like is **word of mouth**. Ask parents in day care or play groups who they use. After that, I advise parents to call the local hospital and ask the pediatric staff whom they might recommend. This gets you started when you are new to an area. It may be necessary to interview several groups to find a practice that works best for your family, your goals, and your values.

Having a physician who listens to you and understands your wants and needs (these are separate issues!) is, to me, the most important point in selecting someone to provide your healthcare. Having rapport and a good relationship with your healthcare provider is the key to good healthcare.

The next information I like for parents to know is how the office works. The nuts and bolts are office hours, after-hours phone calls, emergency care, payments, and prescription policies.

I have discovered through the years, that in order to see a provider who really listens to me and really helps my family heal, it is worth driving a little farther and paying out of pocket.

As in all relationships, communication is the foundation on which to build. I know in my practice I may not always meet the *wants* of a parent, but I will most certainly meet the *needs* of the child for the situation.

I like to explain why certain policies arise or help parents alleviate frustration when things don't run smoothly. There is rarely a time that communication does not resolve a challenge or prevent a potential problem.

Some patients want to know if a doctor is board certified. This is a good question, but just because a physician is not board certified does not make him a poor healthcare provider. Likewise, just because a physician has been sued, does not make him a "bad" doctor. While there is a lot of data you can look up, it is still important to interview a potential physician to get to know him or her and the practice. I know one young mother who had to interview ten practices before she found one doctor who would listen to her concerns about raising her child and help her accomplish her goals.

Immunizations
Do's and Don'ts and Why

The Franz Center is "Pro" Shots

If you examine the history of vaccines, you can see they were born out of necessity, as infectious diseases have been, and continue to be, the number one killer of children worldwide. Most of us have been fortunate to grow up in a time where polio, diphtheria, measles, whooping cough, and rubella no longer cause countless and pointless deaths. Most of us have never seen measles or polio. Most of us have no recollection of the iron lung machines for polio victims.

Most of you have not had a child die from meningitis, nor have you held the hands of a child as he died from this terrible illness. Most of you have never had to tell a family their child would die from an infectious disease like meningitis. Physicians are VERY jaded and opinionated about their view on shots because most of us older than thirty-five remember days and nights when we watched children die from meningitis or invasive pneumonia. Since the implementation of the HIB vaccine in 1985, the incidence of Haemophilus Influenza type B (HIB) meningitis has drastically reduced. Better hygiene has had nothing to do with it.

Polio is projected to be eradicated worldwide by 2010. There was a recent outbreak in 2002 in the Dominican Republic and in Angola. There was also a minor outbreak in Minnesota in an Amish community in 2006. International travel has allowed the threat of many diseases to become a real possibility; look at the books and news information on bioterrorism. Infectious disease secondary to international travel would decimate populations. Thanks to SARS we now know it takes eighteen hours for a virus to traverse the globe. Just because we have not had any problems in the U.S. does not mean there could not be a problem from international travel in the future.

If I had a grandchild at this point, I would immunize the way I immunize my patients. No more than two shots are given at one time. Patients are watched closely for any adverse reactions. I could not live with myself if my grandchild contracted an illness and suffered long-term damage or death from an illness for which there is an acceptable vaccine.

I do not think vaccines are all goodness and light either. Some children with very sensitive immune systems do not tolerate vaccines and can suffer long-term health issues after vaccination. The challenge is that we do not know who they are before the vaccine is given.

In my opinion, our best screening information at this time is the family history. We ask for an extensive family history, three generations back, on both sides of the family (of the mother and father *of the child*), aunts, uncles, and cousins, etc. This is critical! It is important to determine if any close relatives had any bad reactions to vaccinations. We also like to know if there is any family history of autoimmune illnesses like diabetes, rheumatoid arthritis, thyroid problems, asthma, lupus, etc. It is important to learn about your families' medical histories to the best of your ability! There is some speculation that a strong family history of autoimmune problems might make some individuals more susceptible to having an adverse reaction to vaccinations. If there is a history that Mom was exposed to heavy metals, then there are health risks to the baby as heavy metals easily cross the placenta!

Our immunization schedule is arranged to cover the meningitis diseases first. The HIB and Prevnar vaccines have the least side effects, in my experience. We give no more than two shots at a time, but up to three or four vaccines depending on the combination vaccines available. Thimerasol has been removed from vaccines.

We do not begin Hepatitis B (HBV) until after nine months of age, unless there are specific risk factors—Mom has hepatitis B or there is exposure to someone who is engaged in high-risk behavior.

Because of the media coverage linking MMR and autism, we do not give the MMR until age two. While there is no scientific proof of a link between these two elements, I choose to believe there may be a connection (I believe it is the number of vaccines given at the same time that begins the negative domino effect leading to Autistic Spectrum Disorder). Because autism, as a naturally evolving disorder, will be evident MOST of the time by age two, we choose to use this age as our benchmark. We feel that delaying this vaccine until two years old gives any patient developing autistic features time to manifest the process. Almost every parent I have spoken with who has an autistic child has relayed that his or her child suffered developmental regression between eighteen and twenty-four months of age (commonly after the MMR at 15 months of age). We do offer the M-M-R components separately for those who ask. Be aware that there is no scientific proof that separating the components prevents autism. I believe there is some undefined link between vaccines and their potential to trigger an autoimmune event that leads to a cascade of dysfunction in predisposed patients. If we were to QUIT vaccinating, the illnesses for which we give them would increase in a short time, and we would see increased illness and possible death from these infectious diseases. The first step, in my opinion, is being aware. Giving fewer shots at a visit, screening family histories, and listening to parents when they tell us "things are not right" can help prevent permanent injury from vaccines.

We respect the rights of parents to refuse to immunize their children. We do NOT agree with it, but we will not chastise or criticize you. We do have an informed consent that explains what vaccines you are refusing, and what can happen to your child without vaccines. It clearly states that *you, the parent, accept all responsibility for this decision and will not hold us liable for your decision should your child contract an illness for which there is a vaccine that is recommended*. We must be clear on this medicolegal issue.

It is very important for parents to realize that at some point tetanus does become an issue! If your child, who is unvaccinated, receives a puncture wound or a dirty wound, then BOTH a tetanus vaccine AND Tetanus Immune Globulin (TIG) MUST be given within seventy-two hours of the injury. A single vaccine does not provide immunity. Antibodies are formed within twelve to fourteen days after receiving a vaccination, which is the same time for incubation of tetanus toxin. There is no specific treatment for tetanus. It is a painful and ugly disease and a bad way to die.

Whooping Cough or Pertussis (The "P" in the DTaP) is also back on the rise. Whooping Cough is 100% transmissible from an infected person to a non-immune person. The people spreading it are actually immunized adults. There are 800,000 to one million cases of whooping cough in the United States on any given day in adults with a "nagging cough." Pertussis has a high mortality rate in children under age one. For this reason we do encourage the DTaP in children!

This practice maintains the philosophy of no more than two shots at a visit. If a child has a reaction that we consider unacceptable, or you, the parent, feels was of concern, we re-evaluate the vaccine schedule for that individual.

Our view on Varivax has changed as well. While we still believe that chicken pox is mostly a benign childhood illness, the risk of serious life-threatening complications has reportedly increased over the last few years. Flesh-eating strep A, or necrotizing fasciitis, is the current villain. Patients with eczema are at increased risk for complications because of the eczema, and we do recommend the Varivax strongly for patients with eczema! I generally recommend giving it after age three. (It is ideal to wait until after age 5 for this vaccine when the digestive/ immune system is more fully developed). If your child has not had chicken pox (Varicella) by age eight, I recommend getting the vaccine. It is a single dose before age thirteen and two doses thereafter. Since many children begin puberty between eleven and thirteen years old, I like for the Varivax (chicken pox vaccine) to be given by age ten. In my practice, we are proving (by measuring serum antibody titers) that Varivax given after age three confers long lasting immunity. Under two, not so much.

The vaccine is safe. Internal medicine physicians are recommending it for their elderly patients to prevent shingles. These adult patients grew up in the pre-vaccine era and had natural disease. Their immunity has waned as they have aged. So the vaccine is safe even in older patients who have had chicken pox previously. (I would not give it to a child who had chickenpox previously!)

We hope this explains our philosophy on vaccines and the reasons for our beliefs.

Remember that with our schedule, your child is behind on vaccines compared to other pediatric practices! However, even on our delayed schedule, all children are up to date by age three years old. Your child may have to receive vaccines at a visit other than your regularly scheduled well visit. You will be required to pay your co-pay for these extra visits. You still have the choice of giving all four to five vaccines at a visit as recommended by the AAP and ACIP...just not in this practice.

In summary:

1. The Franz Center is PRO vaccines.
2. Our vaccines do not contain Thimerasol except the DTaP and Trihibit, which contain less than 0.3 mcg per dose, which is "Thimerasol free" according to FDA standards. This miniscule amount is apparently unavoidable from the "manufacturing process."
3. The Td or TdaP (for seventh grade) and the flu vaccine (for ages three and up) no longer contain Thimerasol.
4. We will separate the M-M-R at your request.
5. This schedule is different from most other pediatric practices. It takes longer to complete, but in the end, is less traumatic for the child and the parents. And by age five and entry to school, the children are completely and safely vaccinated.
6. This slower schedule will not affect your child's attendance in day care.
7. If you transfer to another practice, you will, of course, be "behind" in immunizations.
8. This schedule minimizes side effects of immunizations and avoids the remote chance of autism related to vaccines (even though there is currently no evidence that autism is linked to vaccines).
9. With this schedule, your child may receive shots at a visit other than your scheduled well-visit. You will be required to pay your insurance co-pay for these extra visits. MMR is also a live virus vaccine and is Thimerasol-free.
10. Rotateq is the new oral vaccine for rotavirus diarrhea. It is given at two, four, and six months. The Franz Center currently does not give this vaccine.
11. If you receive vaccines at your local health department, the staff there often tries to scare parents or bully

them into receiving ALL the recommended vaccines. You have a right to vaccinate your child slowly. If anyone tries to scare you simply stand your ground. You may receive two vaccines or none. You can always go back.

12. DO: get vaccines slower.

    DO: your research

    DO: pay attention to your child's response to Vaccinations

    DO: be your child's advocate

    DO: communicate your concerns to your Physician

    DO: be aware that your child will be fully immunized by age five whether vaccines are given according to the recommended schedule or the slower (safer) schedule.

    DON'T: be bullied into compromising what is important for your child.

    DON'T: be afraid to stand up for you beliefs.

    DON'T: give more than two vaccines at a time.

AAP / ACIP Immunization Schedule

2 months	Prevnar / HIB / HBV / DTaP / IPV/Rotateq
4 months	Prevnar / HIB / HBV / DTaP / IPV/Rotateq
6 months	Prevnar / HIB / DTaP /Rotateq
9 months	HBV
12 months	Varivax / Prevnar
15 months	MMR #1
18 months	Trihibit / IPV
4 yr.	DTaP/IPV / Varivax #2
5 yr.	MMR #2
12 yr.	TdaP/ Menactra /Gardasil (for females)

Immunization Schedule

No Daycare			Daycare
2 months	DTaP #1 /HIB #1	Diptheria, Tetanus and Acellular Pertussis	DTaP #1/ Prevnar #1
4 months	DTaP #2 / HIB #2	HIB- Haemophilus Influenza type B	DTaP #2/ Prevnar #2
6 months	DTaP #3 / HIB #3	Prevnar = for strep pneumonia	DTaP #3/ Prevnar #3
9 months	IPV #1 / HBV #1	IPV= Inactivated Polio Virus	IPV #1/ HIB #1
12 months	IPV #2 / HBV #2	HBV= Hepatitis B virus	IPV #2/ HIB #2
15 months	IPV #3		IPV #3
18 months	HBV #3/ Trihibit	Trihibit= DTaP #4 and HIB #4	HBV #1 / Trihibit
24 months	Prevnar #1		HBV #2 / Prevnar #4
26 months	MMR #1	MMR= Measles Mumps Rubella	HBV #3 / MMR #1
36 months	Varivax #1	Varivax= Chickenpox (Varicella)	Varivax #1
48 months	DTaP #5 /IPV #4	live virus	DTAP #5 / IPV #4
60 months	MMR #2	Varivax #2 or serum levels for antibody titers	MMR #2
		for Varicella and MMR can be drawn as proof of immunity	

- Varivax can be given anywhere between 3 years old and 8 years old to obtain long lasting immunity
- M-M-R can be separated and will need three separate visits after age two to complete
- First Prevnar given at age two requires only one vaccination for immunity
- First HIB given at 15 months requires only one vaccination for immunity
- If a Varivax booster is required between ages 4 and 5 it is best given with DTaP or alone and not in combination with MMR
- The vaccine schedule can be rearranged or vaccines substituted depending on availability of vaccines. It can also be tailored to the individual child's needs.

There are new vaccines being recommended at adolescence now. The Td (tetanus booster) is changing to a TdaP, adding a safe form of Pertussis-whooping cough to boost immunity in the adolescent population.

Rotateq is the "new and improved" oral vaccine for Rotavirus, a very nasty diarrhea infection. It must be given between two months and six months of age. It can be given no later than eight months of age. While Rotavirus is a nasty infection and the number one cause of death from dehydration in third-world countries, I feel the parameters are too narrow. It must be started by six weeks of age, and the last dose cannot be given any later than eight months. I do not give this vaccine in my practice. While it may be a decent vaccine, there are still too many vaccines too early, in my opinion.

Rotavirus diarrhea can be severe enough to require hospitalization and IV fluids. Thousands of children contract this diarrhea each year and a handful of these children will need IV fluids, which resolve the problem.

We currently do not recommend routine vaccination for Hepatitis A either.

At the time of this publication, A Varivax (chickenpox) booster has been added to the schedule. It is recommended between ages 4 and 6 (assuming your child was vaccinated at age one). It seems that one vaccine, given under age two, does not consistently confer sustained immunity. In my practice, if the vaccine is given at age 3 or older, I would recommend a chickenpox titer before school entry. If negative, I would suggest the booster, as we still do not want teenagers and adults at risk to contract the illness. If positive, your child has sustained immunity and does not need a second shot!

Recommendations also include the Menactra—a shot to protect against meningococcal meningitis. This is an uncommon but deadly form of bacterial meningitis that presents like the "flu" but progresses rapidly to death. I describe it as "it looks like the flu and you go to bed and die eight hours later." It is most prevalent in dormitory/barrack situations like college or military living. The media is marketing to eleven-to-fifteen-year-olds. I still believe that it is best administered at the end of high school (or any time your child will be living in crowded situations) when your child is going off to college to live in a dorm. If your child lives at home or in an apartment, then contracting the illness is less likely.

The Gardasil, to prevent cervical cancer from HPV (Human Papilloma Virus), is being marketed heavily to teenage girls and is being recommended at the eleven-to-thirteen-year-old well visits. I have had several patients who have had bad reactions to this vaccine. I have huge ethical issues with giving a vaccine to a young adolescent without educating her on how to prevent this disease. Educate her—don't have sex. I believe that educating and instilling values can decrease the incidence of the human papilloma virus and cervical cancer by reducing early sexual activity. If a female patient is ready to engage in sexual activity, then the vaccine should be discussed. For me, it has too many negative aspects to recommend wholeheartedly.

Below I have included a vaccine record for you to use. Fill in the dates each time your child receives a vaccine(s). Your own permanent record is important.

You may write the age of your child in column B and then the date of the shot.

All vaccines currently recommended are listed. Your child may not receive all of them depending on your physician's practice and your choice.

An excellent resource for further reading about vaccines is Dr. Bob Sears, *The Vaccine Book.* You can find more information on his website at www.thevaccinebook.com, as well as by ordering the book.

The following is a clear visual of current recommendations and how vaccines are given at The Franz Center.

While this is an easy to follow schedule, vaccines can be substituted and given in any order as long as there are not more than two given at a time.

Also visit our website www.Franzcenter.com

	HIB	PREV	DTaP	IPV	HBV	MMR	Rota	Measles	Mumps	Rubella	Varivax
1 mo											
2 mo	✓	☺	✓				Not giving				
4 mo	✓	☺	✓				at				
6 mo	✓	☺	✓				This time				
9 mo			☺	✓							
12 mo			☺	✓							
15 mo	✓			✓							
18 mo		✓	✓		☺						
21 mo			✓		✓						
24 mo		☺			✓	✓		☺	☺	☺	varivax
27 mo					✓			☺	☺	☺	can be
30 mo								☺	☺	☺	given
33 mo								☺	☺	☺	anytime
36 mo				✓				☺	☺	☺	between
39 mo											age 3
42 mo											and 8
45 mo											for sustained
48 mo			✓								immunity
60 mo						✓		Titers	Titers	Titers	

* Happy Faces indicate places where vaccines can be substituted or other times they can be given

Vaccine Record

DtaP			**RotaTeq**			
DtaP			**RotaTeq**			
DtaP			**RotaTeq**			
DtaP						
DtaP			**Varivax**			
			Varivax			
Hib						
Hib			**Fluzone**			
Hib			**Fluzone**			
Hib			**Fluzone**			
			Fluzone			
IPV						
IPV			**Gardasil**			
IPV			**Gardasil**			
IPV			**Gardasil**			
HBV			**Menactra**			
HBV			**Td or TdaP**			
HBV						
Prevnar			**HepA**			
Prevnar			**HepA**			
Prevnar						
Prevnar						

Name: _____

DOB_____

Chapter Two

Watching Your Wonderful Child Grow

Newborns

Welcome to the brave new world of parenting! A world of constant change and joy...the joy of watching your child grow and change. It is also a world of occasional frustration and sleepless nights—problems that come with the territory.

We are here to help you raise your child, not to tell you how to do it. In this office, the physicians and nurse practitioners (ARNP) share the staff and the office equally. All are well trained, and we share the same values. Each of us has our own individual approach to medicine, but overall, we practice with the same goals in mind—quality care for you and your family.

I no longer make rounds in the hospital. If your child needs hospitalization, a hospitalist will provide the care as an in-patient and then you will return to our office after discharge. This has worked very well since its inception. The hospitalists are colleagues of mine, and they are extremely thorough and trustworthy. Hospitalist care for the inpatient is becoming a nationwide practice. Ask your pediatrician about hospitalists in your community.

At the Franz Center, well-patient appointments can be made with the provider of your choice, but it is essential that you see all the providers to become acquainted. When you need an appointment because your child is sick, we will schedule it with the first available healthcare provider. If you specify a preference, we will do our best to accommodate you, but realize that it is more important that your child be seen in a timely manner. The earlier you call in the day for a sick appointment, the more likely you are to see the provider of your choice. Our system works to decrease waiting time and to ease the anxiety that arises when your child is sick.

Winter time is our busiest season, and there are days where wait times are undesirably long. We give each child the time he or she needs, and if the child is really sick and needs admission or extensive testing, it takes extra time to care for him properly. We know that each of you will appreciate the extra effort if your child is the one in need, so we appreciate your understanding when it is someone else who is in need.

Regular Appointments

After your newborn is discharged from the hospital, please call the office for an appointment. We like to see newborns for the first time within three days after discharge from the hospital. Regular checkups follow at two months, four months, six months, nine months, twelve months, fifteen months, eighteen months, twenty-four months and yearly after that. Because we are booked six to eight weeks in advance for well-appointments, we encourage you to schedule your next appointment as you leave the office.

We do our best to meet your **needs** when you schedule an appointment. Sometimes we have to make special arrangements to get your child seen. We appreciate your patience in helping us work with you

Telephone Calls

Telephone calls can be helpful in caring for your child. Phone calls are a form of communication and not a means of diagnosis. There is no substitute for a face-to-face visit. Please do not ask us to diagnose over the phone. Standard practice today is to see a patient BEFORE any medications are given. No one calls in prescription medicine without seeing a patient anymore. Our nursing staff is well trained and can answer most of your questions. When you call, please give the receptionist a brief description of the problem. The call is then triaged by the nurse. Sometimes a nurse cannot answer a call right away because she is busy with patients in the office. Someone will get back to you as soon as possible. We encourage you to write to us via our email: franzcenter@aol.com or fax us at 407-857-7099. The healthcare providers prefer the fax and e-mail whenever possible. The fax and e-mail are a more direct form of communication from you and can contain more detail than we often get on the phone. The fax/e-mail is then given to the providers and a direct response is written back to you.

The healthcare providers do not return calls during business hours. It may take one to two days for a healthcare provider to return patients' phone calls. Your best bet is fax, e-mail, or an office visit to receive a quicker response.

After-hours phone calls are for problems that cannot wait until the office reopens. Our calls are handled by Tele-Kids, a service staffed by knowledgeable RNs. They follow strict protocols and all information is documented and faxed to us the next morning. If they cannot address your problem, the MD or ARNP on call will be contacted. **There is a charge for the after-hours service.**

Payment

Be sure that you add the baby to your insurance *before* your two-week visit. Insurance companies do not automatically add your infant to your policy. We allow two months for your insurance to pay on filed claims. After that, it is your responsibility to straighten it out with the insurance company and pay your balance.

General Characteristics of Your Baby

Being born is as physically traumatic for the baby as it is for the mom. Thus, your newborn may have some transient and peculiar physical findings.

Head

The head may be *molded* or *misshapen* from the journey through the birth canal. This molding usually subsides quickly, but may take one to two months to resolve totally. The child's scalp may have a collection of fluid called a "caput." This results from the passage through the birth canal and disappears quickly. There may also be bruising of the face and head. These problems are normal and disappear quickly.

Eyes

The baby's eyes may be puffy for a few days. They may have a yellowish discharge that results from the eye drops used at birth to prevent blindness from infection. Drainage that appears five to twenty days after birth may be the result of a blocked tear duct or an infection. Both are common problems and are easily cared for with eye drops and massage.

Skin

The skin may be dry and flaky. It is often worse in post-term babies. Babies can slough the first layer of skin, like a snake, for up to three weeks. You can use lotion on their skin. It really does not help the peeling, but it will not hurt them, and it often makes Mom feel better because she is doing something. Their skin can also develop several "newborn rashes" that can come and go over the first several weeks. They can have *milia* or "milk bumps." Newborns can also develop a fleabite looking rash all over the body that comes and goes. These fleeting rashes are normal, need no treatment, and disappear after a few weeks.

Remember, when babies get cold, their skin will take on a blotchy purplish color. This is normal.

Chest

Many infants develop breast enlargement with possible milk drainage during the first few weeks of life. This is a response to their mother's hormones and disappears spontaneously. There is also a noticeable bump on the chest of many babies. It is the end of the sternum; the xyphoid process, and it becomes less noticeable as the baby grows.

Legs and Pelvic Area

The legs appear bowed in all infants. Their feet may also turn inwards. These characteristics are a normal result of being folded up in utero. These characteristics disappear and the legs straighten out as the infant grows.

In girls, mother's hormones are also responsible for vaginal discharge. Withdrawal of hormones after birth can lead to blood-tinged vaginal discharge in a baby girl. This is not a reason for concern, and it stops after a couple of days. It is not heavy like a period.

Cord

The cord is ugly but functional. It falls off one to two weeks after birth. Clean the cord with alcohol once a day. During other diaper changes, clean with a Q-tip and water. Skin germs are necessary to debride the cord, and if you use alcohol with every diaper change, the cord area remains too clean, and the skin germs cannot do their job efficiently. Too much cleanliness delays cord separation. When it does come off, the umbilical area can ooze, stink, and bleed for up to seven to ten days. Just clean with alcohol and water as before, and this will stop.

Birth Weight

All babies lose weight the first few days after delivery. They can acceptably lose up to 10 percent of their birth weight in the first three days after birth. They regain the weight quickly. Average weight gain in the first month is one ounce a day. Some infants can gain as much as two to three ounces a day in the first few weeks. All weight gain is excellent. Many infants have poor appetites initially, but they catch on quickly once they become hungry. If you are worried about your child's weight gain, the best thing to do is make an appointment. We do not recommend a scale at home to weigh your child, as this tends to shift mothers' focus from feeding to weight checking.

Remember your child just experienced labor and delivery. It is a *relief* to be born, and we are asking this person to adapt swiftly to a new world of things! Some infants need time to adapt and rest up after all that hard work.

Jaundice

Some babies develop a yellow skin color called jaundice. Jaundice peaks between days three to five after birth (hence part of the reason we want to see your baby during this time). In utero, the environment is relatively low-oxygen, and the placenta does the majority of detoxification work. The baby in utero makes extra blood to help stay oxygenated. Once born, the baby needs to take over these functions, and the liver does the work of detoxification. Because the lungs now work, and the environment is rich in oxygen, there is no longer a need for extra blood, so it is broken down into a product called bilirubin, which is stored in the fatty organs of the body. The two biggest fatty organs are the skin and the brain. A certain level is considered normal, and excessive levels (greater than twenty-five) can potentially damage the brain. So, if your baby is really yellow, we will obtain a bilirubin (bili) level and start phototherapy if warranted.

Amusing Activities

All newborns make funky noises. They sneeze, cough, gag, hiccup, whoop, and cross their eyes. As long as the baby eats well, stays pink, and is otherwise fine, these amusing antics are of no concern. Babies must breathe through their noses when they are eating. If they can eat well even while sounding congested, it is no problem. If the baby cannot eat because of the congestion, that is a problem, and the baby needs to be seen. Many of these noises are made as the baby tries to clear his or her nasal and chest passages.

Stools

All newborns grunt and strain as if pooping is a national incident. They make noises that sound like a truck driver—no malice intended for you truckers. The baby will draw up his legs and strain. This is annoying, but normal. As long as the stool that is passed is soft and mushy, no interference is needed. Initially, babies pass thick black tarry green stools, called meconium. Then the stool becomes brownish-yellow, and finally yellow and/or seedy.

Breastfed babies produce very thin liquid orange yellow stools. They may occasionally have green stools, and they may poop initially up to twelve times a day (after every feeding). These are not diarrhea stools. After two to four weeks, the frequency will reduce to three to six times a day, and by two months, in an exclusively breastfed baby, the stools may be as infrequent as once a week. That once-a-week poop can fill three to four diapers! What a load!

Bottle-fed babies produce stools similar to breastfed babies except their stools are usually a bit thicker (more like Play-Doh). Bottle-fed stools can be brown, green, and yellow. The only unacceptable stool colors are snow-white, blood-red, and pitch-black. If your child has a stool that is one of those unacceptable colors, a visit to the office is needed. Bring a sample of the stool with you. Bottle-fed babies generally produce stools every day to every three days. Constipated stools are rock hard round balls that are difficult to pass. Call our office if your baby is truly constipated.

Sometimes there is blood in a baby's stool. There are several causes for this, all of which are usually simple and benign. A small streak of blood can be caused by tiny tears in the baby's anus. These tears are called anal fissures. Sometimes milk, either milk-based formula or excessive dairy intake in the breastfeeding mom's diet, can cause an allergic reaction that causes irritation and inflammation of the colon and leads to blood in the stool. Taking milk out of the baby's diet usually resolves this problem.

DO NOT PANIC! Fortunately, blood in the stools is not dangerous or life-threatening.

If there is more blood than stool coming out of the baby's rectum, this is a problem. Please call for an appointment. If it is after hours, please go to Night Lite Pediatrics, After Hours Pediatrics, or Arnold Palmer Emergency Department (or in your area, the nearest hospital providing pediatric emergency services).

Birth Marks

Birth Marks are very common, and interestingly, many show up a few weeks after birth. Common areas to find birth marks are the nape of the neck, over the eyelids, and on the forehead. The technical name is "strawberry nevus" or "flame nevus." I have also heard them called "stork bite" or "angel kiss," and they fade with time. They are formed from tiny capillaries near the surface of the skin.

Some children have a ***nevus sebaceous*** on the scalp somewhere. These often look like an orange peel. They will need to be seen by a dermatologist around the age of six. They are not a concern in newborns.

Crying

Crying can be good for the baby. It is never good for the parents. It is important to remember that it is a form of communication from your child, as she does not yet have language. Parents quickly learn to differentiate a "wet cry" from a "hunger cry" and from a "hurt or frustrated cry." Often, there is no clear reason for the crying. Some infants simply need to let off steam, and they may have a fussy time of day. Popular hours for this fussy time are between 4:00 and 7:00 p.m. (commonly known as Arsenic hour, and many families do not answer the phone during this time), 10:00 p.m. to 12:00 a.m., and then anytime after midnight. It is okay to let the baby cry for a little while to work out his frustrations. It is okay if Mom and Dad cry too. It helps detoxify your system.

Soft Spot

The anterior fontanelle or soft spot is the area of the head where the head bones come together. There are seven cranial bones that are not fused at birth. This allows them to move and expand. Many newborns have ridges that are prominent where the sutures actually overlap. In time, they move themselves into a nice, round shape. There is no need to worry. The soft spot is usually flat, but it may be slightly bulging in a normal baby. It also will pulsate. This is normal. You cannot hurt the soft spot unless you actively try. We do not recommend trying. The soft spot may be bulging and tense when the baby cries, and it may be sunken a little when the baby is quiet.

Feeding

Feeding is obviously important. Babies do not grow if they do not eat. Feeding time is a pleasurable time for the infant, as well as quiet bonding time for the mother and baby or for the father and baby.

Nutrition is very important throughout our whole lives. Whether you choose to breastfeed or bottle-feed, your baby will get everything she needs. Formulas and breast milk provide all the right ingredients for your child to grow.

Do not be confused by ads that say you should feed this or that at a certain age. A lot of that is marketing. The formula that is right for your baby's early months is good until she is twelve months old. If you think you want to make a change, please talk with your provider first.

We encourage you to feed your baby on demand. "On demand" is usually every two to four hours. The amount taken may vary from feeding to feeding. Burping relieves the baby of excess air. However, not every baby burps after feeding.

Some do not swallow a lot of excess air. If your child has not burped after five minutes, do not keep trying to force it out of him. Put the baby in a "baby bouncer" which has the baby at a forty-five degree angle of elevation. Then put the baby with his right side down. This position helps promote self-burping. The gentle pressure of being put on his tummy can also help the baby burp.

Breastfeeding moms will find their milk comes in about three to four days after delivery. You can get your milk to come in faster by feeding the infant every thirty minutes to an hour for one to two minutes at a time. This frequent feeding the first day or two for a few minutes at a time brings your milk in faster. It helps reduce engorgement, stimulates uterine contractions, and prevents nipple soreness.

Many moms worry that their baby is starving until their milk comes in. This is not so. Colostrum, which is the thick yellow "first milk," is rich in antibodies and growth factors that the baby needs. If

God meant for milk to be in at delivery, it would be so. Colostrum is the perfect initial food for your child. Colostrum contains more protein, fat soluble vitamins, and minerals than mature milk. It contains less calories as well. Colostrum provides 67 kcal/100 ml where mature milk is 75 kcal/100 ml. Breast milk contains fat, carbohydrates, and protein. Fat comprises 50 percent of the calories in human milk. The protein is primarily whey protein, and in cow milk, the protein is casein.

Some babies need a short resting period before they figure out that breastfeeding is fun, and some take to it straight after birth!

There are five basic steps that help breastfeeding go well.

First, Mom must be comfortable with her arms and back supported.

Second, position your baby so his or her body is tummy-to-tummy with you. The ear, shoulder, and hip will then be in a straight line with the areola.

Third, offer the breast with your fingers under the areola with your thumb resting on top, at least an inch away from the areola. This position gives the baby access to pools of milk behind the nipple.

Fourth, have the baby latch onto your nipple correctly by waiting until his mouth is wide open, then pulling him in fast. The nose should be touching the breast but not occluded by the breast. If it feels like you are smashing her into the breast, you are doing it right. The baby can breathe. Lift with your fingers under the breast to move the breast away from the nose—do not push down from the top of the breast.

Fifth, break suction with your forefinger before taking the baby off, or it will really hurt.

Infants need eight to twelve feedings a day in the first week. Feeding more during the day will mean less feedings during the night by the time she is a few weeks old.

We do not recommend supplemental feeds with formula or water during the first two weeks, provided the baby is nursing well and gaining weight. Studies have shown that babies who are bottle supplemented too early may experience nipple confusion and lose more weight. Babies supplemented too early can also regain weight more slowly. Occasionally slow gainers need supplementation!

For moms who do not like milk there is good news! Breastfed infants whose mothers do not eat many dairy products develop fewer allergies and less eczema. Therefore, milk restriction can be beneficial.

For working moms, new information shows that if you breastfeed for one month, you will protect your baby from lower respiratory illness for several months. Four months of breastfeeding is considered optimal for protection against lower respiratory illness and allergies in the first year of life. Breastfeeding until age one is ideal, but not every mom can, and not every baby wants to. It is great to know that breast feeding for one to four months offers healthful benefits. Getting some breast milk every day, even if it is pumped breast milk, helps a lot to protect your baby from allergies, asthma, eczema, and infections.

Long-term studies are showing that breastfeeding, or breast milk pumped, can offer protection against infant diarrhea, RSV (Respiratory Syncitial Virus), strep pneumonia, Haemophilus Influenza, eczema, ear infections, celiac disease, childhood cancer, diabetes, SIDS, and obesity. Asthma rates are lower in children who are exclusively breast-fed in the first four months of life.

The hormone prolactin causes milk production, and the hormone oxytocin causes uterine contractions. Frequent breast-feeding stimulates uterine contractions and lessens post partum bleeding. There is speculation that breast-feeding may decrease osteoporosis, as well as the risk for breast and ovarian cancer.

Breast-feeding is uncomfortable initially, but that should get better within the first two to four weeks. The new onset of filling and emptying of the breasts can cause some discomfort (duh!).

If you have bleeding, cracking, scabbing, or pain during a feeding, please call the office. We also have two excellent lactation consultants in this area to whom we refer!

Infants generally nurse five to twenty minutes per side per feed. Some prefer to nurse one breast, fall asleep, then awake in an hour to nurse the other breast. Some just nurse the one and are done. If you are really full and uncomfortable, I recommend pumping the full breast. I never liked leaving a full breast until the next feed. It hurt, and I hated being lopsided. During the first ten minutes, the baby gets 90 percent of what she needs. The last 10 percent is hind milk, which is rich in fat. This hind milk helps the baby gain weight and be able to go longer between feeds. Babies often will nurse longer in the mornings and evenings to compensate for longer intervals at night. My children never nursed longer than seven minutes a side. They are strapping teenagers now. Do not fret if you have a short nurser who is nonetheless still gaining weight!

Working mothers can continue to breast-feed after they return to work. We will discuss options with you on one of your visits, or you can discuss it with a lactation consultant. Breast-feeding mothers need to drink plenty of fluids to keep their milk supply plentiful. You should also eat a balanced diet. Eat anything you want; the key is to eat in moderation. Foods that are known to cause problems include dairy, nuts, and spicy foods in particular. Lesser culprits that can cause problems include chocolate (I have *never* believed this, but I have read it somewhere), caffeine, cabbage, broccoli, asparagus, citrus, and tomato stuff. You do not have to necessarily avoid these foods; just pay attention to any problems that arise after you have eaten them. This means the baby will be miserable after you eat certain foods, so avoid them. Drinking beer or wine (one glass—no boozing it up) is okay, as it relaxes Mom and helps the letdown reflex.

There are a few medical reasons not to breast-feed:

1. If the mother has active tuberculosis, she should not breast-feed until she and the infant have been treated.
2. HIV infection in the mother.

3. Mothers with herpetic breast lesions.
4. Mothers receiving chemotherapeutic agents.
5. There are only a few medications that prevent breast-feeding. Examples are nuclear medicine isotopes, some antibiotics, immunosuppressive agents, and lithium. We have reference resources to consult when there is any concern about a mother's medication and breast-feeding.

Bottle-feeding is not that different from breast-feeding. Both involve giving the baby a nipple and then milk comes out. (I went to medical school to learn that.) Anyway, the baby should still be fed on demand. Formula is heavier in consistency than breast milk, but has the same number of calories (twenty) per ounce. Babies stay satisfied a little longer on formula (three to four hours vs. two to three hours). The average newborn takes one-half to one ounce initially but can quickly work up to two ounces a feed every two to four hours in the first week. Bottle-fed babies tend to be greedy and eat quickly. They can overfeed, meaning they take in more than their stomach can hold. When they overfeed, they simply vomit the extra. It is helpful to burp the greedy baby after every ounce consumed to reduce air in the stomach and gas after the feed. This may not work with some infants, as they will simply scream when being burped because they prefer to be eating. This screaming causes more gas. In this situation, it is simply better to feed the baby and then burp him. A little wet burp is nothing to worry about. Your choice of formula can vary. I still prefer *Similac*™, *Enfamil*™, *and Prosobee*™. WIC currently offers Good Start products only. *Gentle Ease*™ is a partially hydrolyzed formula. It is a wonderful balance between milk-based formula and the totally "pre-digested" formulas. It seems to reduce gas and fussiness in many babies. *Lactofree*™ is for those who are lactose intolerant. Thus, there are many choices and sometimes it takes a bit to find the right one for your infant. It is important to know that about 30-50 percent of children allergic to the casein in cow's milk will also be allergic to soy protein.

Vitamins and Fluoride

Find out if the water in your area has had fluoride added to it. OUC (Orlando Utilities) does add fluoride. Orange County Utilities does not. If your water is fluoridated, you need do nothing. If it is not, or you have a water purifier, consider using fluoridated bottled water or adding fluoride drops to the diet. Fluoride really helps build strong teeth. I do not push it unless there is a family history of bad teeth, or there are other circumstances that demonstrate your child really needs it. Fluoride is tricky. The right amount is perfect. Too little predisposes to cavities, but too much can permanently discolor the permanent teeth. You do not know if it is too much until the permanent teeth come in. I apply common sense to the situation.

We do not routinely recommend multivitamin supplements to infants. Breast-feeding moms taking their prenatal vitamins will supply the baby with vitamins. Formulas contain vitamins. Premature babies, poor eaters, or breast-fed infants who do not start solids until six months may need supplementation. The literature says that after four months all babies should have a vitamin supplement. God gave me two boys who hated everything supplemental. Getting vitamins in them was a battle. I decided a good relationship and harmony in the house was worth more than following literature recommendations. I made sure they ate well, that I ate well, and that I took my vitamins. That worked so much better for me! They are still alive and doing well.

Vitamin D is the newest of insufficiencies in our diet, and vitamin D supplementation is now recommended. If you live in an area where vitamin supplementation clearly makes a difference, <u>or you believe your child will benefit from extra vitamins, then supplement!</u>

Cleaning Bottles

If you own a dishwasher, you can safely wash your bottles and bottle nipples in it. Water temps above 120 degrees provide adequate sterilization. If you do not own or use a dishwasher, we recommend sterilizing bottles and nipples until the baby is two months old. After that, hand washing or dishwashing is okay. After two months of age, you can quit using sterile water to mix the formula.

Solid Foods

I think solid foods are good. There are so many tasty things to eat and try, especially if you know a good chef! For babies, we recommend starting solids after four months of age. Formula or breast milk provides all the nutrients the baby needs initially. Early introduction of solids, before four months, increases the risk and probability of food allergies, obesity, and excess salt intake. Interestingly, introduction of foods after six months also increases risk of food allergy. Ideally, solids should be introduced between four and six months of age.

You may begin with whole grain rice. Rice helps maintain the digestive system and improve immunity. After rice (and mush it as much as you need to), introduce veggies and fruits that are generated from a flower on the plant. Peas, green beans, beans, tomatoes, eggplant, and squashes, all come from a flower. So do "fruits" as we think of them. Introduce one new food every three to seven days. This way you can see if your child is sensitive. If so, you can actually dilute food to 1/6th and introduce it that way (Like a weak soup).

Clothing

No special precautions need to be taken in dressing your child. The house should not be too warm or too cold. Common sense tells you this. Whatever you are comfortable in, the baby will be comfortable if dressed in similar weight clothes plus one-layer lightweight clothes when it is warm and heavyweight if cold. You can make a baby too warm and give them "bundle fever." So if you are happy in T-shirt and shorts, your baby will be miserable in a winter sleeper with feet and a blanket!

Be sure the baby does not sleep in a draft. Ceiling fans are a must in Florida. It is fine to have one on in the baby's room but not blowing directly on the baby. It can make the baby cold, but will not cause a cold, according to the research.

Bathing

Bathing the baby in a tub is not recommended until the umbilical cord falls off. Sponge baths are fine until then. Newborns do not need frequent baths. Maybe one or two a week will be sufficient. Skin creases should be clean and dry. If left damp, the creases are prone to develop yeast rashes. Yeast rashes are bright red. The genital area on little girls should be gently wiped from front to back. Do not rub. The cheesy substance that seems stuck there forever will disappear slowly with gentle cleanings.

Diaper Rashes

Diaper rashes are common in infants. They can occur at any time and are not usually a reflection of poor care of the baby. Diaper rashes are rashes in the diaper area and can be of several types. Generally, just good hygiene and over-the-counter ointments will resolve the rash. Desitin, A&D, Balmex, Dr. Flanders, Bag Balm, Calendula, Aloe Vera, and Triple Paste are all brands that can be used. These are not the only ones we recommend. If you have one that you love, and it works, use it. These are all over-the-counter (OTC) brands. Air and water are also good "lotions" for your baby's skin. If a rash is not improving after three days on one of the above ointments, the rash might be a yeast rash. Tinactin, Micatin, Gyne-Lotrimin, Monistat, and Lotrimin are over-the-counter creams that can help. A diluted solution of EITHER vinegar and water or baking soda and water can help get rid of the rash. This diluted solution can be used every diaper change to clean the baby. Mix one teaspoon of vinegar or baking soda to one cup of water. Vinegar OR baking soda both help break up cell wall membranes of the yeast. Beyond this, if the rash is not going away or is pustular looking, the baby needs to be seen.

Umbilical Hernias

Umbilical hernias are protrusions of the belly button, or "giant outies," as we call them. These hernias are common. They are the result of a hole in the abdominal wall where the placenta was attached. They typically are as big as a fingertip of someone with small hands. Umbilical hernias spontaneously resolve by the time the child is three to five years old. They can be ugly and disturbing to look at, but they are not painful and do not cause problems. If the hernia hole is bigger than two fingertips, or the hernia does not improve by the time your child is three years old, then surgical repair may be needed. Putting a quarter over them or a truss makes you feel better but does not help the hernia go away faster.

Crowds

Fear of crowds is called agoraphobia, but that is not what this section is about. Babies should not be in crowds until after eight weeks of age. They should not be in the malls, supermarkets, at family reunions, or in church. If your baby is born during the fall or winter, I am adamant about no crowds for eight weeks. The reason is simple. The baby's immune system is initially the same as the mother's immune system. Any new viruses or illnesses mom has not had, the baby can contract. The infant immune system can be overwhelmed with illness, and infants can become critically ill in a short period. ALL infants under the age of four weeks who develop a fever are AUTOMATICALLY admitted to the hospital and started on IV antibiotics until the cause of illness can be determined. I have maintained in my practice that it is not worth the risk to expose your infant to crowds in these first eight weeks of life. Of course, the family is excited and everyone wants to see the baby, but if this child becomes ill, who pays for it? You, the parents, pay for the illness financially, emotionally, and psychologically. Relatives and friends can wait until it is safer for the baby to be out in crowds.

There are always special circumstances like weddings, funerals, and christenings. We can discuss those special circumstances on an individual basis and figure out how to accomplish what you need while keeping the baby safe.

Circumcision

Circumcision remains a bit controversial. The AAP recommends not doing it. However, it is a personal decision and if you want it done then it is best to have it done in the hospital before discharge!! The pendulum is swinging more towards circumcision again. Recent studies show there is a definitive decrease in AIDS and penile cancer in the circumcised male.

We no longer do circumcisions in the office. The hospitalists will do them prior to discharge and as an outpatient.

There are two basic methods of circumcision—the plastibell and the gomcko. The plastibell stays on for seven to ten days and falls off on its own. There is no routine care after this procedure. The more common method, and the one the hospitalists use is the gomcko. With the gomcko method, the foreskin is removed and then it is necessary to put Vaseline on the penis for seven to ten days until it heals. Both methods provide symmetric and aesthetically appealing results.

Do not worry about the method of circumcision. One is not better than the other. ANY procedure is only as good as the doctor performing it, and our experience has been very positive! The hospitalists do numb the penis area before the procedure, so it is no longer a painful experience for the baby.

Elective circumcision is done in the newborn period. After the newborn period, a urologist or pediatric surgeon must perform the procedure, and the child needs general anesthesia. The surgeons in our area do not do elective circumcisions. Circumcisions are done beyond the newborn period <u>only if</u> there is a medical indication.

Well, this covers most aspects of newborn care. Enjoy the baby. Your instincts and basic common sense will keep you and your baby safe. There really is too much information available and it can make you paranoid and neurotic. I recommend not reading a lot of books. I like *What to Expect the First Year* and *Baby 411* as resources. When friends and family offer advice that is phrased, "Let me tell you what worked for me," then it is wise to listen. When it is offered as, "Here is what you <u>have</u> to do, or here is what you <u>should</u> do," I generally do not listen. Every baby is an individual, and what worked for one may not work for another. Experience is a great teacher, especially the experience of those you trust. When others tell you how to raise your child, they do not account for the nuances and individualization of you and your family. That information is likely not to be helpful, may be confusing, and may even cause you frustration.

Two-Month visit

Your baby is two months old now. He/she is lifting her head with more control, following your face from side to side, and smiling and cooing on purpose.

Hopefully she is sleeping through the night, but it is normal for a two-month-old to be up at night one time between 10:00 p.m. and 6:00 a.m. A breast-fed baby may still be eating every two hours during the day or every two to four hours around the clock. Many breast-fed babies at this point also decrease the frequency of their stools, going as little as once a week. But when they go they will fill three to four diapers. This is normal! Pooping patterns will even out when you introduce solid foods sometime after four months of age.

Bottle-fed babies can take as much as four, eight-ounce bottles per feed. Baby boys tend to eat a lot more than baby girls do. Eating up to thirty-six ounces in twenty-four hours is normal. For some children, if they are eating forty ounces of formula a day, we might suggest the introduction of solids (cereal only) to ease the financial drain of that much formula.

Many infants really begin to become "porkulent" which is healthy. We do not worry that they will be fat later. Many pile on the weight until six months old and then "grow into it." We do not put infants on diets. Their brains are being fed also at this time.

I generally discourage the use of goat's milk as an alternative at his age, as infants we have tried this with in the past have not grown well. Raw goat's milk is also deficient in folic acid.

Your baby will receive his/her first set of immunizations today. We only give two vaccines at a time in this practice. It is my belief that their immune system can handle only two at a time. In addition, do you remember reading anywhere in history that people got all these diseases at the same time? After shots, a knot in the leg, low grade temp. (100-101) can be expected. Generally, because vaccines are really improved these days, we get very few reactions. Those we do get are not bad. You can never tell who has a sensitive system before shots are given. If your child seems unusually ill after shots, call our office during regular office hours.

Safety begins now. Do not put your child in his car seat on any counter. They can catapult themselves unexpectedly off and be injured. Do not trust them for even a second on a bed or changing table, as again they can surprise you when you least expect it and roll off.

By your next visit at four months, your child will laugh out loud at you (I love that sound), blow raspberries, babble more, bat at objects more purposefully, and hopefully sleep all night.(Defined as 2200 to 0600) No solids until after four months (except as above if taking more than forty ounces. a day.)

Your child will receive two more vaccines at four months which are the same ones he received today.

_____*and* _____

*Ht.*_____ *Wt.*_____ *HC*_____

Four-Month Visit

Your baby is now four months old, much more entertaining and a lot more fun. He/she is laughing out loud, blowing bubbles, batting at things more on purpose, and sleeping better.

Some babies roll over one way at this age. Rolling both ways is a six-month milestone. Your child might be sitting for a few seconds in a tripod position (a six-month milestone). Most babies have doubled their birth weight by four months. Your child can lift his/her head and chest up off the table now.

If you are ready, you can consider starting solid foods at this time. You can use baby food or table food. I recommend table food. The general rule is if you can mush it, then he/she can try it. Introduce one <u>new</u> food every three to four days. If there is a strong family history of allergies or food sensitivities, then introduce food at six months or present one <u>new</u> food every seven days. Begin with rice. Whole grain rice helps nourish and maintain the digestive system. If you want to do a cereal, we recommend Earth's Best cereal. Then move to fruits and vegetables. The trick is introducing foods <u>that grow from a flower on the plant. This includes many traditional fruits as well as foods we consider vegetables</u> like peas, green beans, peas, acorn squash, butternut squash, winter squash, eggplant, tomatoes, and all beans, etc. Use fresh or frozen veggies. For fruits, use fresh or natural. (Bananas and mangos are not best first foods because they hinder digestion). Pears or peaches by Libby's packed in their own juice are fine if you want to use canned fruits. You can use Mott's Natural Applesauce. You get the idea. Plums are great as are nectarines. Pineapple should be cooked first. This makes it sweeter and healthier for babies. If you introduce a couple "veggies" (ones that grow from a flower as mentioned above) first and then sweet fruits, your child will not prefer the sweet all the time. My motto is simple, "If you can mush it, your child can eat it." The mushing removes lumps a child can choke on. Use these "fruit" foods until twelve months. Then introduce vegetables. Vegetables are literally considered the <u>other</u> edible parts of plants including roots, tubers, leaves, stems, and bulbs. So non-flowering vegetables are introduced ideally at twelve months. (Carrots, potatoes, sweet potatoes, spinach, broccoli, cauliflower, beets, etc.) Corn can be allergenic so waiting until after age one is excellent.

Meats are best introduced after twelve months as well. Eighteen months would be ideal.

Occasionally a baby will get constipated when you start foods. If this happens, we suggest P-FRUITS: peach, pear, plum, prune, papaya, pineapple, pumpkin, and peas. P-fruits make you poop! You can use the actual fruit or the juice. We do not recommend juices as a regular part of the diet because they are empty calories. But for constipation they are great!

It is not necessary to start with cereal. You can just use rice. For some babies, cereal can be allergenic or constipating. In this case, move right to "fruits" as described above. Use a spoon, not an "infant feeder." Sit the baby up for feeds, not lying down. You can feed once a day or gradually increase to three meals a day. Follow your instincts and the baby's desire and readiness.

I suggest looking at the Hallelujah diet as it has some useful suggestions. I do not myself buy into all their philosophy, but have found some useful ideas for introducing a healthy diet to your child. I have provided healthy ideas. If you vary your methods and your child is doing well, no worries.

Once you introduce foods, your baby might want less formula or decrease a breast feed per day. This is normal. After all, we are introducing them to more calories so they will naturally want fewer from the bottle or breast.

At four months, your child CAN sleep from 10:00 p.m. to 6:00 a.m. If he/she is not, you have the choice of getting them to sleep all night. For 99 percent of children, letting them cry it out will solve the problem. For many mothers, this is a challenge. The maternal instinct has us thinking we are hurting them somehow or scarring them for life. NOT TRUE.

The first step is in initially putting them to bed. Develop a bedtime ritual—reading, rocking, and singing, or whatever you like. When the child is "drifty," that stage where you can tell they are getting ready to drop off and their eyes flutter, put them in bed. Of course, the baby will pop up as if to say, "Hello, I am not asleep." You can pat his/her back gently until he/she falls asleep. The first night it might take thirty minutes. If need be, get a kitchen timer and set it for thirty minutes the first night. Then twenty-five the second, twenty the third and so on until you are in there less than five minutes. After that, it takes less and less time. But this way when the baby wakes up at night he/she will be able to put himself back to sleep. What bliss!

When they wake up in the middle of the night, let them cry for five minutes, and then check to make sure they are okay. Do not feed them. They really are not hungry (assuming we are already feeding solids. If not, then I suggest feeding them solids in the evening). Checking every twenty minutes helps you get through this time while not giving in to the baby. The first night is usually the worst and subsequent nights are better. Your actions say, "I hear you, I understand, and I empathize. Now deal with it." This philosophy will actually help you through the next eighteen years. It is not a requirement that you "make" your child sleep all night at this age. But the advice will be the same no matter what age you choose to help your child sleep all night.

(These techniques I learned from Dr. Ferber's book, <u>How to Solve Your Child's Sleep Problems.</u>)

WARNING! If you as a parent do not feel you can do this, then don't. We have lots of time to solve this challenge.

By next time (six-month visit) your child will sit in a tripod position for three seconds or more, transfer things hand to hand, squeal because he/she can, bounce on his/her legs when you hold him up or in Johnny jump up/"exersaucer." Many six–month-old babies are on all four's rocking. A few are crawling. Most are rolling over both ways and roll all over the house.

We do not recommend walkers. Studies clearly show that babies in walkers are more prone to injuries. If you have one, take the wheels off so the child cannot be mobile in the walker. Keep small objects out of baby's reach. Anything smaller than the baby's fist is considered a choking hazard. Begin thinking about baby proof tactics now. If you have a pool, be sure you have it fenced off!

<u>Drowning is a preventable accident!</u>

Your child will receive two more vaccines today (the same ones as at the two-month visit).

_____ and _____

Ht_____ Wt_____ HC_____

Six-Month Visit

Your baby is now six months old. He/she is rolling over both ways, sitting up in at least a tripod position, squealing, babbling, and hopefully sleeping all night. This is a great age for the "johnny-jump-up" or "exersaucer." We do not recommend walkers, as they are too dangerous. If you have a walker, take the wheels off so the baby is more stationary. Studies also show that babies in walkers have delayed locomotor development (crawling and walking). Think about it, why propel yourself if you have a vehicle that you can maneuver faster! Don't forget to use car seats all the time in the car.

If you started solids at four months, then your baby might be up to three meals a day. Remember that many babies on solids will decrease their formula/breast intake a little bit. Not to worry. If you are still using baby food, go ahead and start table food. If you can mush it, the baby can eat it. Rice or pasta, (cooked, of course) is okay to start. Green beans, peas, winter squash, peas, pears, plums, beans,

applesauce, etc. are all good foods to introduce one at a time at this age. (See four month visit on feeding). I generally do not recommend starting meats until after a year or until your child can take table food, fruits and veggies. After one introduce the root vegetables like carrots, potatoes, beets (which nourish the blood and prevent anemia). Dairy, wheat, corn, and nuts are the four most allergenic food groups. Avoid these as well as citrus. No honey until after age one. Berries are very healthy and can be introduced one at a time at this age: Blueberries, strawberries, raspberries, and blackberries. Occasionally children will have a local reaction around the mouth to one of the berry family. If so, just wait a while longer to introduce that one. Berries help repair DNA.

Many six-month olds are very chubby and parents often ask about this. Babies are supposed to be a bit chubby. They grow into it as they begin to "exercise" by crawling and walking. There is nothing wrong with being lean either. What did you and the baby's father look like at this age?

You can begin practicing with a cup. It is a new skill and they are not going to be coordinated at first. That's why we say "practice." If your baby is formula fed, then be sure to put formula in the cup on occasion. Watered down juice, water, Gatorade are all okay to use in the cup. Juice is a dessert food to us. You may start it, but water it down. Most juices are empty calories and contain too much sugar. So use them diluted for variety.

Be sure the house is baby proof and poison proof at this time. If you have a pool, be sure it is fenced off so baby cannot reach it.

If your baby is not sleeping all night, revisit the four-month visit instructions.

Your child will receive two more vaccines today.

_____ and _____

Your next visit is at nine months of age. Your baby will learn to get on all fours and rock, pull to a stand, perhaps cruise around on furniture, and (for some unfortunate parents) your child will be walking! They are into everything when they walk so early (But, oh so cute). Some are able to wave bye-bye and clap or bang things in the midline. Your child can sleep all night at this point. They will babble more and even say "Mama" and "Dada."

Ht_____   Wt_____   HC_____

Nine-Month Visit

Wow! Your child is really growing and becoming more and more independent. By this age, most children can sit alone. Some can right themselves if they fall to the side. Some can get from a lying to a sitting position. Many are crawling, pulling to a stand, and cruising furniture. Some are walking! Your child may bang things in the midline (clap), and even throw some things. He/she likes to take everything out of cabinets. Some can wave bye-bye, and some are saying "Mama" and "Dada."

At this point, your child <u>can</u> sleep all night. Refer to the four-month visit for details. If you have tried those suggestions, we recommend Dr. Ferber's book, <u>How to Solve Your Child's Sleep Problems</u>.

If your baby is still on jar foods, graduate to table foods. In general, we recommend waiting until one year of age if possible to introduce meats. Continue formula or breast-feeding until age one. We do not suggest changing to regular milk before then. At this point, your child should begin or be on some solid foods. Also continue to practice with the sippy cup. If your nine month old can drink from a straw, that is even better than a sippy cup, according to an oral motor therapist I know. Be sure to put formula or milk in the cup to have your child get used to milk in a cup. Some babies think milk=bottle and bottle=milk and when you want to wean the bottle, they will not drink milk. While this really is okay, it can be avoided by introducing formula in a cup in these "practice" stages.

It is time to be sure the house is "baby and poison" proof. Do not leave your baby unattended. They can drown in a bucket of water or a toilet. They are becoming more curious. This is a good time to create a "Tupperware" cabinet—a cabinet with plastic dishes the baby can take apart and play with without fear of injury. This way they also do not make a lot of noise with these dishes. Never leave your child unattended. (This bears repeating many times!) They can get into danger very quickly. They experience their world and learn through sight, sound, touch, taste, and smell. They love electrical outlets, toilets, and anything that is remotely dangerous.

If you have a pool, be sure it is fenced off!

Today your baby will receive two more vaccines. _____ and _____.

Your next visit is at twelve months. Your child will be walking alone or very close to it. Your child will wave bye-bye, bang midline, say two words we understand (Mama and Dada), and be into everything!

At twelve months, we also do a screen for lead and anemia. This is a finger prick or can be a venous draw. Your insurance requires you to have this done at a lab of their choice. We will provide you with the prescription for it. This is especially important if you live in an old house or a new house that is under five years old.

Ht_____ Wt_____ HC_____

Twelve-Month Visit

Can you believe it has been a year already? Can you believe the incredible changes that this person has made? He/she has learned new motor skills and learned a language…okay, learned to understand a language. By age one, your child can walk alone or be close to it. Some children are very cautious and wait until they can get it just right. They all walk by seventeen to eighteen months, and if they do not, we get a physical therapy consult. Many children (more boys than girls) will have a "clumsy" stage about three months after they begin to walk. They stumble on air, trip over invisible toys, and walk into walls. This can be very bothersome. It is normal. I believe their brain is faster than their body, and they have a wiring gap that is only temporary.

At this age, you can switch from formula to whatever milk you drink— 2 percent, or whole milk. Skim milk is not acceptable, as it does not contain enough fat for brain development. NO milk is an acceptable alternative as is soymilk, rice milk, and goat's milk. It is actually a good idea to introduce soy, rice, and regular milk, so your child is used to all the tastes, and you have an option. Of course, if your child is allergic to soy or dairy, don't introduce all of them. Your child should be on primarily table foods. It is best to avoid peanut butter until two years of age. Almond butter and the like are fine. Honey is fine after age one.

Your angel CAN sleep through the night. It is normal if your child has been sleeping through the night for him/her to begin rousing in the middle of the night from teething or dreaming. After six months, children's sleep patterns begin to be more adult like, and they dream. It is a normal developmental milestone.

From twelve to fifteen months, discipline is primarily through distraction. "NO" is for danger or things that are "no" under any circumstance, any place, or any time. Children this age respond to exchange; trade them one item for another. If you say "No" to every little thing, they quit listening sooner, and not listening happens all too soon and persists for years!

If this child is second or more in line, then he or she might be faster or slower in development than his or her siblings might. Often, subsequent children want to catch up and be like the older sibling. Other times, he or she figures the older sibling is pleasing the parents with all his or her abilities, so this child will hang back and take things at a more relaxed pace!

Today your child will receive two more vaccines: _____ and _____.

If you have a history of exposure to TB or anyone in your family has a chronic cough, your child may need a PPD—a tuberculosis skin test.

We also recommend getting a lead level and hemoglobin (for anemia) at this age.

Your next visit is at fifteen months. Your child will walk alone or run alone, say two to five words, imitate, throw temper tantrums, sleep all night, and be OFF THE BOTTLE. After fifteen months, the bottle increases potential for ear infections and cavities. The best way to get off the bottle is to take all the bottles your child receives in a day, and wean one bottle a week. Many babies will not take milk in a cup unless you began that practice before now. Their minds' associate bottle= milk. Milk=bottle. So if it is in a cup, they refuse it. This association is easy to solve. Stop the bottle and all milk/formula for two to four weeks. Out of sight, out of mind. Then reintroduce milk in a cup. Breast-fed babies don't use this rule.

Ht_____ Wt_____ HC_____

Fifteen-Month Visit

Welcome to toddler world, where everything is fair game and the adults have to keep their eyes open and senses keen. Your baby is now mobile. Some are walking, and some running. Most are climbing.

Most can say two to five words. Some say no words. However, if your child understands a lot and babbles with inflection, then we can be assured this child can hear. Some children choose to store up words in their brains until they can speak in full sentences. We are not concerned if a child is saying no words until eighteen to twenty-four months. Children in bilingual households will often be a bit slower in expressive language, and when they do speak, it may be a mixture of the two languages.

Your child is eating and probably becoming a picky eater. Most children over the age of one eat one good meal a day, and generally, it is not for the parents! He/she will not starve! Children are intuitive and eat what they need. They often eat in spurts, as well. One week your child may eat beans; the next applesauce; and the third week, meat. Over three weeks, he/she will eat a balanced diet. Children often love something for two weeks and then won't touch it after that. That's normal. A lot of children slow down their weight gain around now. That's normal. Some children stop gaining weight altogether. We will discuss that at your visit. A nice little trick for the picky small child is to put one teaspoon of vegetable oil (I prefer olive oil) in the food three times a day. This adds good fat and calories and can beef up a poor eater's diet.

Children at this age can sleep ALL NIGHT. Many begin to wake up again from teething and dreaming. Do not feed them and start a bad habit. Your child should be off the bottle (or VERY close). Pacifiers can stay until eighteen months. Getting off the bottle is the first priority.

You may begin to give your child choices. This cultivates independence and lets him/her feel empowered. The choices are simple and concrete—this cup or that cup, this toy or that toy, this shampoo or that shampoo. "My way or the highway" is a choice. As the ADULT, you are in control of the big choice. For example, "We are going to take a bath, but you can choose your shampoo and towel. We are going to get dressed, but you can choose your pants." (You get the idea). Failure to make a choice is also a choice, and then it reverts to the parent to decide. Ah, the power of choice!

Today your child will receive one or two vaccines:
_____ and _____.

Your next visit is at eighteen months. Your child will run, climb, talk, and be able to perfect all his/her skills. Temper tantrums begin or accelerate. IGNORE them and they diminish. Promise. Your child will increase his vocabulary by doubling the number of words between fifteen months and eighteen months.
Your child will be off the bottle and sleeping all night. In addition, most children are eating three meals a day in some fashion.

Continue your bedtime ritual. Children thrive on structure and routine. Repeated patterns of behavior help form brain circuitry. This is why they read the same book 12,000 times, eat the same food for two weeks at a time, and watch the same video until you want to scream. It is helping them form brain circuits needed for development. This is one reason why learning to be consistent in discipline is so important.

Say what you mean and mean what you say. Being consistent and following through on consequences is very important in setting boundaries. If you cannot or will not follow through on a consequence, do not make the threat. Let the child suffer the consequences of his/her own behavior.

In the real world, every action has a consequence, GOOD or BAD. If you follow the rule, you stay out of trouble. If you don't, you suffer the consequences. This begins now for your kids. Watch how they manipulate you with those big sweet eyes and sad little voice that says, "I sorry. I not do it again." It's a TRAP. Don't fall for it! Of course, they'll do it again! They are children! So we learn to say, "I love you, and I believe you, but the consequence stays in place." Then you get the temper tantrum. Oh, these beings are skilled! But we are still the adults and really do know what is best for now.

Ht_____ Wt_____ HC_____

Eighteen-Month Visit

Isn't this child the cutest person you have ever met? So smart and constantly amazing you every day! It just keeps getting better from here. At this age, your child should be walking, running, climbing, throwing tantrums, sleeping all night, eating one to three meals a day, and sleeping all night.

Your child should be OFF THE BOTTLE. Once off the bottle, it is time for Mr. Binky (the pacifier) to find a new home. I recommend this around eighteen to twenty months. The most efficient way to stop the pacifier is to cut the end off and give it back to the child. This way it is "broken," and they give it up voluntarily. A few will want to hold onto this for awhile. That is okay. It can stay in their bed and be a comfort at night. But this way, the parent is not the bad guy. I highly encourage you to eliminate the pacifier before language skills are good. You do not want to hear, "Take me to the store, and buy me a new one." There are some eighteen-month-olds who can do that!

Temper tantrums should be flourishing or on the way. Ignore them. Begin brushing teeth to the best of your ability. Some children want this. Some hate it (mine did). If it is a challenge to brush their teeth, you have a choice. I had to sit on my first one, pin his arms with my knees, and gently pull his hair to open his mouth. Then I brushed his teeth. Now this is not something you want to do all the time. So the next time, I sweetly asked, "Do you want to brush your teeth, or do you want Mommy to do it?" He did it. See, it's all about choices. Give them constructive choices.

Say what you mean and mean what you say. Being consistent and following through on consequences is very important in setting boundaries. If you cannot or will not follow through on a consequence, do not make the threat. Let the child suffer the consequences of his/her own behavior.

In the real world, every action has a consequence, POSITIVE or NEGATIVE. If you follow the rule, you stay out of trouble. If you don't, you suffer the consequences. This begins now for your kids. It can be entertaining to watch how they manipulate you with those big sweet eyes and sad little voice that says, "I sorry. I not do it again." It's a TRAP. Don't fall for it! Of course, they'll do it again! They are children! So we learn to say, "I love you, and I believe you, but the consequence stays in place." Then you get the temper tantrum. Oh, these beings are skilled! But we are still the adults and really do know what is best for now. (Yes, this is repeated from fifteen months...)

Your child will receive two vaccines today:
_____and_____

Your next visit is at two years of age. By then, your child will jump on two feet (both feet come off the ground), talk in two to four word sentences, and throw temper tantrums. Some count to two, and some know one or two colors. At two, they can recognize "Show me the blue ball, etc." but cannot answer, "What color is this?"

Terrible twos is a real entity. They recognize they are separate from you and have learned the power of "NO" and "MINE."

They are independent and want to do things themselves. Encourage that within reason. They also go through a phase where "No" means "Yes." Learn to be creative with your language. Instead of saying, "Don't do that" which guarantees they will do exactly the opposite, try, "If you do that then this will happen." For example, "If you touch that, you will get burned. If you play with that, you will get hurt." This really works. Of course, do not let them do anything that would be dangerous or result in a trip to the ER! Boys more than girls really need this kind of experience. Control the outcome! Let them experience the results of their actions within reason!

Ht_____   Wt_____ HC_____

Twenty-four Month Visit

Welcome to the world of the two-year-old. Things really do not change for the next eighteen years—language just improves! Now your toddler can talk in two to four word sentences, jump off the ground with both feet, throw temper tantrums, and scribble. Many know eight body parts, walk backwards, count to two, and know one or two colors.

Your child should be off the bottle and the pacifier. Your child should be sleeping all night. Terrible twos is a real entity. The two-year old recognizes he/she is separate from you and has learned the power of "NO" and "MINE."

They are independent and want to do things themselves. Encourage that within reason. They also go through a phase where "No" means "Yes." Learn to be creative with your language. Instead of saying, "Don't do that," which guarantees they will do exactly the opposite, try, "If you do that then this will happen." Example, "If you touch that, you will get burned. If you play with that, you will get hurt." This really works. Of course, do not let them do anything that would be dangerous or result in a trip to the ER! Boys more than girls really need this kind of experience. Control the outcome! Let them experience the results of their actions within reason.

As parents, say what you mean and mean what you say. Pick your battles. Be consistent with the issues that matter. As parents, you need to agree on what needs discipline, but you do not necessarily have to discipline the same way. Different children respond to different methods of teaching. Personally, I am a "counter." I have always counted to three. This gives the child time to "regroup" and change his/her behavior. By the time I reach three, there is a consequence that follows. "Time-out" is a valid consequence and is a minute-per-year, or two minutes for a two–year-old. There is controversy over whether you should use the crib as a time-out place. If you remember the purpose is to "regroup," then the crib or child's room is a safe place to do so. Even if they have fun in there, as long as their behavior changes, then the method worked.

You can also consider putting your child in a "big boy bed" (or "big girl bed").

I suggest putting the crib on its lowest setting, removing the sliding rail, and putting up a Fisher Price guard rail. It is forty-eight inches long and fits most cribs. Simultaneously, put a regular twin bed in the same room. (I think the toddler beds are a waste of money because children outgrow them so quickly. Also the guardrail is not for use on toddler beds). Let your child play on the twin bed, nap on it, and become familiar with it. After one to two weeks, take down the crib, and move the guardrail to the twin bed. Push the bed against the wall, so the wall serves as the other "guard rail." Once your toddler is in a twin bed, he/she will crawl out. Tell your child at a non-discipline time that he/she must stay in the room. If he or she does not, then you will put up a gate. If the child climbs the gate, you will close the door. If she can open the door, then you will lock the door (after you have turned the handles around so you can lock her in). You will open/unlock the door when she stays in the room. You will have to follow through. Once your child knows you mean business, then she will stay in the room. If you find your child sleeping at the door threshold, that is okay. She is in her room! This does not damage children because you have explained the rules ahead of time, and it is not cruel because you will open the door when they stay in the room.

For those who have trouble with this concept, you can allow them to come into your room when they have climbed out of bed. HOWEVER, they can sleep only beside your bed on the floor. Do not make it comfortable for them! The object is for them to be cold and uncomfortable, so they will choose to stay in their own room! For the small subset of kids who will wander the house and possibly get hurt, stick to the first plan.

Many children between two and six will also have nightmares and/or night terrors. With nightmares, they cry and wake up. They are consolable. Night terrors are more frightening. Children cry, sleep walk, and have their eyes open, but they are not awake. Night terrors seem to occur at about the same time every night. Do not try to wake your child; just put him back to bed. Night terrors seem to occur with stress (like a long day at Disney, or a sibling picking on them, etc.).

If night terrors are frequent, and you see they are about the same time each night, then go into the room about fifteen to thirty minutes before they usually occur and gently disturb the child's sleep state. Rouse them to groggy. Do this every night for seven nights, and that should stop the terrors. The homeopathic remedy Calcarea Carbonica 200c can also effectively end them. Give 2 pellets dissolved in an ounce of water nightly for seven nights.

<u>Potty Training</u>: Most children begin to show interest or signs of readiness at this age. At first, it as simple as telling you their pants are messy or wet and need changing. Boys are slower than girls. In general, do not push toilet training. They own this! You can do all kinds of things to people, but you cannot control when they poop and pee. I do not believe in bribing, potty songs, or books. I have found the best way to achieve this milestone is to be patient, non-judgmental, non-critical, and to have no expectation! I do not know of any children who have gone to Kindergarten not potty-trained. My recommendation is to begin at two years, four months (I arbitrarily picked that age.). Many families have another baby at this time, and the baby needs to be four months old before you begin anything with the first child). Then from SUNUP to SUNDOWN you take this child potty every two hours. It is tedious, but it works. DO NOT ask if the child has to go potty. You just go. You try. Sometimes you will have success, but most of the time not, initially. It takes about a month before they get the hang of it for pee. Poop comes later. I told my kids that it was important not to hold their poops in. I would rather they go in their pants than hold it. I was willing to provide a diaper for that sole purpose if they desired. This is a short-lived stage. You can try the big potty or a potty-chair. Every child is different. When they went poop, I would take them in the bathroom, flush it, and tell poopy bye-bye. I would say, "This is where poop goes." I felt this was important, as many children are afraid of the big toilet. They identify somehow with their stools and think they will be flushed as well. By dumping poop out of the diaper in there with them present, I felt it desensitized their fear and made it all logical.

Most kids accomplish potty training between two and three. If they are a bit later than that, do not worry!

Your next visit is at three. By three, your child will stand on one foot, talk in bigger sentences, throw tantrums, count to ten, sing ABCs, and be-oh-so much smarter.

If your child is behind on shots, then you will receive one or two today. If up to date, then the next shots are at age four.

Ht_____ Wt_____ HC_____

Vaccine _____and_____

We recommend Varivax (chicken pox vaccine) at twenty-seven months or later, but by age 10.

Why age ten, you ask? Well, when my son was ten years old (and he had had chicken pox at age three), I looked at his beautiful skin and thought I would not like him to get chicken pox at that age or later and have his beautiful skin poxed up.

Chicken pox in the adolescent and adult age group is a worse illness with more scarring and increased chances of getting secondary complications, like pneumonia or strep infection of the lesions themselves.

Three-Year Visit

We can only hope it has been a whole year since we saw you last. And what a year it has been. Your three-year-old has successfully weathered the "terrible twos." If your twos were benign, then threes will be a challenge. Now little Miss/Mr. Chatterbox talks your head off and puts concepts together that amaze you.

Discipline concepts remain the same. Say what you mean, mean what you say, and follow through. Set appropriate boundaries and stick to them. Pick your battles, be consistent, and avoid power struggles. Children thrive on routine and respond to boundaries even when they act like they don't!

After age three, we recommend the big push on safety (for every visit hereafter!). Begin with body parts. Tell your child the correct name for his/her privates and who can look. The correct answer is usually Mom, Dad, and when he or she goes to the doctor. Adjust it for different family members as you see fit. Generally, aunts, uncles, and grandparents have no real business seeing private parts unless they are routine caregivers. Talk about good touch and bad touch, and what to do if someone does touch them in a way they don't like. Encourage communication, and teach your child there is no shame. Just get the facts.

After age three, your child can go to the dentist. We can recommend a pediatric dentist if you need one.

Almost all children become picky eaters at this age. I get hundreds of questions on this subject. Fortunately, the answer is always the same. If your child has convinced you that he/she will only eat chicken nuggets from McDonald's, it is your fault. (This actually happened to me with one of my own children. It was a rude awakening!) Make a big sign, and put it where you can see it all the time. It should say, "I AM THE ADULT." I have had to be reminded many times that I am the adult. The children should not be running our lives. It is meant to be the other way around. Now our parents were right. Eat what Mom or Dad cooks or go hungry. Do not run a restaurant at home. You are providing good nutrition for these children. IT IS

THEIR CHOICE NOT TO EAT. If they choose not to eat, they go hungry. Soon they will get the message and eat what you give them. I really leave no room for negotiation on this subject. Children will not starve to death, but they will manipulate you to death if you let them. It is frustrating as a parent to go through this, but persevere. The rewards are great. There is an old saying you can begin to use. If you like to eat, learn to cook. If they do not like what you cook, they can learn to cook. Now this is not actually practical for a three-year-old, even up to ten or eleven, but it makes a point. When they say, "But I am too little," they are right. So eat what your parents cook. Provide them with fruits, veggies, protein, and grains. After that, it's up to them! It is not acceptable to say, "I don't like that" when they have not even tried it. It is not necessary to clean their plate, but it is necessary to try what is on it. Do not let food be an issue for you as parents. You provide it. They eat it. If they do not, no dessert or bedtime snacks. It is simple. No argument, just choices with consequences.

After this age, I recommend you add the words, "it's your choice" to daily conversation. Every action has a consequence, good or bad. They get to choose how they want to behave and hence choose the consequence. If they choose to misbehave, then they choose what you offered. This is powerful and helps reduce the frustration and anger we feel when we have to discipline them. I have made these mistakes for you. I can tell you that consistency, boundaries, and detachment really work! Detachment means not being attached to their behavior. The best way to see this is to imagine disciplining someone else's child. You see the bad behavior, and you provide straightforward boundaries and follow through. You can see through their manipulative behavior and provide kind, firm rules that they respect and respond to. It is amazing how all that objectivity flies out the window when the child is yours! God has a funny sense of humor.

If your child goes to day care, be clear on who will pick up your child every day. Develop a code word so your child knows what adults are safe. Role-play "What would you do if so-and-so came to pick you up? Would you go?" Asking questions that encourage your child to think and respond really helps you see how they are processing information. There are no wrong answers. If you ask a question that should clearly have a "no" answer ("Can a stranger touch your privates for a new toy?") and you get yes, then you know your child doesn't understand yet, so you spend the time educating. This is a repetitive process for the rest of your lives here! The car is a great place to ask questions about safety. It is nonthreatening, and you get the most interesting information from them. Ask age-appropriate questions, and those relevant to your own life circumstances. Because our children have two medical parents, they know a whole lot more about trauma than other children. We always explained fairly exactly what will happen if you continue to do that behavior.

(Ex: if you run with a stick in your mouth, it will perforate your soft palate, sever your carotid artery, and you will die before I can call 911. This approach works for my kids. It may not work for yours, so adapt it).

You will hear a lot of the same information from here on. Values and safety do not change; we merely upgrade it to meet their age-appropriate needs.

If you like to read, here are some of my favorite books.

1. Raising a Son and the sister book Raising a Daughter by Don and Jean Elium.
2. How To Talk So Kids will Listen and Listen so Kids Will Talk by Faber and Mazlich.
3. Secrets of the Third Pig by Charlene Messenger.
4. 1, 2, 3 Magic by Thomas Phelan.
5. Redirecting Children's Misbehavior by Kvols and Riedler.

There are many more terrific books on raising children. I like the practical approach. We all make mistakes, but learning to apologize and admit when we make mistakes—while remaining firm and kind—is a great way to raise great children

Ht_____   Wt_____

Four-Year Well-Visit

Four is a great age. Actually, they all are great ages with their strong points and their drawbacks. But at four, your child can hop on one foot, skip, talk in large volumes, know his colors, and can count to fifty (or close to it). I hope that your child has learned to swim (especially if you have a pool in the backyard). Your confident self-assured four-year-old is beginning to challenge you a little. This is great as it means you have raised this child to be safe and secure enough to have the confidence to challenge you. Now we must rein it in.

Discipline concepts remain the same. Say what you mean, mean what you say, and follow through. Set appropriate boundaries, and stick to them. Pick your battles, be consistent, and avoid power struggles. Children thrive on routine and respond to boundaries even when they act like they don't.

If you have a picky eater, refer to the three-year visit. Basically, eating should not be an issue. It has boundaries like other behavior expectations. You eat what is in front of you; you try new things when requested, and if you choose not to eat, okay. You can eat at the next meal, and there are no snacks later. If our children are really picky eaters, it is sad but truly our fault. So detach from it, and let it be his/her choice to eat the good food you have prepared. Yes, I like vitamins and other supplements, but the word "supplement" means "in addition to" not "instead of." So while supplements will help bridge the gap in nutritional problems, continue to work on getting your child to EAT a variety of foods. Mannabears and Yummi-Bears are good supplements as they contain the equivalent of four ounces of vegetable juice. Also, Juice Plus™ is an excellent supplement containing all the phytonutrients in fifteen fruits and vegetables and two grains. New studies show that the "gummi" vitamins increase the risk of cavities. I love gummi vitamins because so many children like them. If something tastes bad, a child will not take it. So, teach your child to brush after "gummies" and that will get the sugar off the teeth and reduce the risk of cavities.

After four, your child should have seen a dentist. If not, make an appointment. Also after three or four, it is nice to see an eye doctor for a check-up, especially if there is a family history of vision problems. Our little eye chart is nice, but it is not the equivalent of a full ophthalmologic exam.

Your child is becoming more and more creative. Encourage creativity while maintaining that he tell the truth as well. This is also a good time to introduce "meditation" or imagery to your child. Children are so much more receptive to these ideas than adults, and these techniques can really help them manage and reduce stress later! My favorite is a bedtime book of visual imagery. Maureen Garth has written three books: Starbrite, Moonbeam, and Earthlight. Any one of them is good. Barnes and Noble Bookstore has them or the books can be ordered for you. There is a prelude for relaxation followed by different scenarios. The guided imagery promotes relaxation, provides a tool for reducing anxiety, and the prelude offers a chance for discussing any worries your child might have. This is an awesome addition to your reading and bedtime rituals. When I started it with my nine-year-old, he asked me after three days, "Mom, are you hyper when you leave my room at night?"
"No, why?"
"Well, that star thing takes all my "hyperness" and relaxes me. I figured all that energy had to go somewhere. I thought you got it."
This was a powerful affirmation that this helped him relax and sleep deeply.

I recommend several books on discipline:
1. Raising a Son and the sister book Raising a Daughter by Don and Jean Elium (the daughter book is twice as thick as the son book).
2. How To Talk So Kids Will Listen and Listen so Kids Will Talk by Faber and Mazlich.
3. Secrets of the Third Pig by Charlene Messenger (I love this one!).

4. <u>1, 2, 3 Magic</u> by Thomas Phelan.
5. <u>Redirecting Children's Misbehavior</u> by Kvols and Riedler.

At this visit, it is time for a booster DTAP. Next year, at five, your child will receive a booster MMR.

Ht_____   Wt_____

Five-Year Visit

Five years is a big age. This year your child will enter kindergarten. He or she can ride a bike with or without training wheels. He or she can tell you his or her address and phone number. She can swim, count to twenty or more, knows the ABCs, and perhaps recognizes some letters. He knows his colors, can cut in a straight line, cut and paste, and extrapolate large concepts.

For boys, this is a big "orifice" oriented age. "Butthead, wiener head" and other attractive phrases enter the vocabulary, almost unbidden. This is normal. It is important to define such words and to teach your child the values of not using language like that. Your basic five-year-old also begins to exert some sassy talk or back talk. This is an important milestone and sets the pace for the next fifteen years. I have become a fan of Tabasco. Soap never worked for me and always made me feel like I was close to abusing my child. But Tabasco has that zesty flavor. It is a food product with nutritious value, and enough of it helps treat intestinal parasites as well. So whenever the mouth has a back talk problem, a dash of Tabasco sets things right. Do not be put off by the precocious child who says, "I like it." Just offer more. Usually a drop on their finger (which must then be put in their mouth) is an adequate solution, but for the child who likes it, a teaspoon or more can be offered. Usually they decline the increased amount.

Safety remains the biggest concern for years. Your child should know how to swim. If he/she cannot, get lessons! We live in a water state with a high frequency of drowning. There is no good excuse for your child to not know how to swim. Anything with wheels can gather speed, so a helmet MUST be worn AT ALL TIMES on a bike, trike, skateboard, scooter, roller blades, etc. The basic rule is simple: "No Helmet, No Bike (trike, scooter, etc) No Discussion." I do not accept the parents' idea that "We didn't have helmets, and we turned out okay. "That is garbage. We also didn't have AIDS, seat belts, high school shootings, etc. Things are different now. Do not live in the past where safety is concerned. You do not want you or your child to become a statistic that defines the need for these interventions! We do not require helmets in the car yet, but a properly fitting seat belt must be worn. Booster seats are recommended until sixty pounds, or age six. Shoulder and lap belts must fit for a safe ride.

Children thrive on routine. Who will take your child to school, and who will pick her up? Tell your child every day. Even if it does not change, she will like the security of knowing. Even at the ages of ten and twelve, my own children liked to confirm if it was Mom or Dad picking them up that day. What time? Tell them who can pick them up and under what circumstances that might happen. Have a code word if necessary. Be clear. Revisit who can look and/or touch privates—Mom, Dad, and when you GO to the doctor. What do you do if someone on the playground shows you his or her privates? (Tell the teacher.) Begin helping them learn how to handle conflict in an appropriate fashion. Boys are physical and believe that punching someone's lights out will resolve most conflicts. Not true. They need to know how to USE WORDS. Even in martial arts, you never throw a punch when words can resolve the issue.

Kindergarten is a huge growth period for you and your child. The emotional trauma of sending your "baby" to school is quickly overcome with the joy of watching him or her flourish as he or she learns. If many kids in his or her class have older siblings, your child will learn much more than you bargained for! Do not get upset. Whatever your child learns, he will share with you. When those bad words come home, explain their meaning at your child's level and why it is not good to say those words(hint:Tabasco). I find that the calmer you are as a parent, then the "taboo-ness" of the word or action is minimized and, hence, no fun. However, if you make a big deal about it, your child will either use it against you to upset you on purpose, or feel shame. We don't want either feeling for your child if we can help it.

Be consistent. Follow through with the discipline you offer. Do not make threats you cannot carry out. Be clear and specific in your explanations. When mine were this age, I would threaten to take away their Game Boy. "Okay," they would say. "You didn't say we lost Nintendo 64, TV or movies." I learned quickly to cover all the bases!

My favorite book for this age and up is <u>Secrets of the Third Pig</u> by Charlene Messenger. It is a great book for teaching our children how to be resilient and offers excellent tips on discipline.

This is a great age for teaching meditation and visual Imagery. We have wonderful books on that as well—<u>Starbrite</u>, <u>Moonbeam</u>, and <u>Earthlight</u> by Maureen Garth are wonderful books for this age and up. They offer a good opportunity for a nighttime ritual.

At five, your child will receive a booster MMR. For those who receive the M-M-R separated we draw blood titers to measure antibodies and prove immunity. If your child has not had chicken pox, I recommend the Varivax. If you are unsure, then I suggest getting a blood test to check for chicken pox antibodies. If positive, no shot. If negative, get the Varivax.

Your next visit is at age six. Everything your child does now, he or she will do better! The journey continues, and you really begin to see the rewards of your labor as well as the traits you hoped he or she wouldn't get from Uncle Harry!

If you have firearms, keep them locked up, and store the ammunition separately. If you do not have firearms, teach your children not to touch <u>any</u> weapons or guns, (except the brightly colored plastic water guns). Do not talk with strangers. Do not let anyone see or touch your privates. Ask them questions, "What would you do if…?" What if someone offered your child a lot of money to see their privates, would they accept? If they say yes, then explain why that is not a good choice no matter how tempting it may initially seem. You can teach without fear or judgment. It works well. Consider there are no wrong answers. Then when your child gives one that scares you, you take a moment to explain why that may not be a good choice.

Now share this next section with your child. I am going to tell him something very important! Your parents WANT to give you privileges. They want you to have everything possible. They love you. You must earn it. You earn it by doing whatever your parents ask THE FIRST TIME. You do whatever they have asked you to do without whining, complaining, or saying things like, "Why can't my sister or brother do it? Why do I always have to? I did it yesterday. Sister (brother) never has to do anything...." Try not complaining and doing what your parents ask THE FIRST TIME for seven days. See how they change and what privileges you earn. I guarantee this works. It's up to you.

Ht_____   Wt_____

Six- to Eight-Year Visit

Somewhere in this time span, the excitement of having children begins to wear off and you find the unwelcome thought on occasion entering your head, "Now why was it that we wanted children?" Is all that I am experiencing normal? Who taught this child that "No" is an acceptable answer to anything I say as a parent? Can I get a refund?

Why must they go to school and learn this stuff? Welcome to the real world of parenting. Now you begin to see the small insights into how your parents raised you (providing you were not the victim of child abuse, abandonment, or neglect), and why they did things the way they did. It all begins to make sense.

Children need structure and discipline. They need to be able to challenge us and know there are boundaries. I read the greatest book years ago. It is called <u>Taking Chances</u> and is out of print now. It was about failure and how important it is to growth. Most of the world's greatest inventions followed on the heels of tremendous failure. Walt Disney was bankrupt eleven times before he achieved ultimate success. Penicillin was discovered as a result of a failed experiment.

Home is the place in which our children experiment and learn what will fly in society and what will not. It seems grossly unfair, if you ask me. It does explain why children seemingly torture us with their misbehavior and act like angels elsewhere. I am also convinced that the more safe and secure a child feels, the more self-confident he or she is, and the more he or she will challenge us. Remember what a grand job you are doing when you are about to pull all your hair out over childhood challenges. It seems, through the years, that the stricter we became and the meaner we felt, the better our children behaved and were more loving. They respect the boundaries and love the attention. They will not admit it, of course.

Safety still is the biggest issue. Continue to educate and explain your rules and reasons for them. As children mature, they dislike our rules more and more; but as long as we continue to explain the reasoning behind these rules, and our fears as parents, children understand. Keep your explanations age-appropriate. They do not need more information than they can absorb.

When your child begins to ask the "tough" questions (like where babies come from, have you ever been in jail, etc., just seeing if you're following here) —stop, take a deep breath, and ask your child, "Why do you ask?" You want to understand the framework for this question. Answer only what the child needs to know. Keep it simple and short. When he wants more information, he will return and ask.

Be sure your child can swim. Reinforce the basic rule: No helmet = no bike, scooter, etc. If you have firearms, keep them locked up and keep ammunition separate. If you do not have firearms, teach your children not to touch any weapons or guns (except the brightly colored plastic water guns). Remind your children: Do not talk with strangers. Do not let anyone see or touch your privates. Ask them questions, "What would you do if…?" What if someone offered your child a lot of money to see her privates, would she accept? If she says yes, then explain why that is not a good choice even though it is tempting.

No shots this year. No more shots until age twelve, unless the gods who decide about shots change the rules.

Now share this next section with your child. I am going to tell her something very important! Your parents WANT to give you privileges. They want you to have everything possible. They love you. You must earn it. You earn it by doing whatever your parents ask THE FIRST TIME. You do whatever they ask you to do without whining, complaining, or saying things like, "Why can't my sister do it? Why do I always have to? I did it yesterday. Sister (brother) never has to do anything…" Try not complaining and doing what your parents ask THE FIRST TIME for seven days. See how they change and what privileges you earn. I guarantee this works. It's up to you.

Ht_____   Wt_____

I recommend the following books:
Secrets of the Third Pig by Charlene Messenger
The Five Love Languages of Children by Campbell

Eight- to Ten-Year Visit

By now, you are well entrenched on the journey from perfect child to unbelievable child. By now, you are beginning to really reap the rewards of good parenting, and you are seeing what your child learned that you had no intentions of teaching him!

Second, third, and fourth grades encompass these years. Your child is learning addition, subtraction, multiplication, and division. He or she is learning to read and write stories. He is also learning history. Guess what? Children are also being taught in school how to follow directions! Third and fourth grades are all about learning to follow directions. This is to prepare the child for middle school. Well, children treat this following directions thing as a class subject. They do not feel the need to do homework or practice this particular skill at home—EVER. There is another course that is self-taught on the playground. This course is how to manipulate parents to jump through hoops. I think it started back in the 50s with the hula hoop. Look how good they are with that and how pitiful we are as adults! *Now is the time to look for common mistruths.*

1. Do you have any homework? No.
2. Did you do your homework? Yes.
3. Did you brush your teeth? Yes.
4. Did you get those school clothes out of the dirty clothes? No.
5. Why is your brother (sister) crying? "I dunno."

Check the homework log. Smell their breath. You can see yesterday's dirt on their "clean" clothes. You know they started whatever conflict with the siblings. Be confident. Take no prisoners. Be clear with consequences. <u>Follow through</u>.

Observe the wily and cunning behavior of this age group. Your children will skate through all rules if you are not aware of their tactics. They know how to work you. Be wise to the big eyed "I'm innocent look." Always accept, "I love you" even when you know they are up to no good.

Advice learned the hard way (These are things worth doing):

1. No TV during the school week.
2. No Nintendo, PS2, Gameboy, Xbox, Gamecube, PS3, Nintendo DS, or any electronic play during the week and certainly not until homework and chores are REALLY done.
3. Be available for a certain time frame each day to help with homework.
4. Continue to dialogue and offer your values. For example, education is important. We expect you to do the best you can. Chores are important to keep the house running smoothly and everyone happy.
5. Bedtime is strict. They will stay up late if you do not enforce it. A tired child is no fun. Continue prayers and your bedtime ritual. The visual imagery of <u>Starbrite, Moonbeam</u>, and <u>Earthlight</u> is incredible at this age.
6. I tell all kids this age that, as parents, we want to give them privileges. We want them to have all they want within reason. Their job is to earn it by doing what we ask them to do the FIRST time. I ask them to actively try this for a week and see how their parents transform. No back talk, no whining, and no blaming someone else. Just do it. See how easy it is to raise good parents with this one simple idea.
7. Kids this age can learn to do laundry, put clothes away, and load and unload the dishwasher.
8. Be very clear about safety. Drugs, alcohol, and even sex can begin to be discussed at this age. Continue firearm safety discussions. Even if you don't have them, their friends' parents might. Lots of families have parents who are police officers or who like to hunt. Answer questions at your child's level. Your children are learning a lot in school and being exposed to lots of information. You want to be the filter and interpreter for them. You want to know what goes on in their world and help them traverse the waters safely.
9. A lot of young girls are beginning menses at age ten. If your daughter is asking questions or beginning to develop physically,

you need to discuss puberty with her. <u>It's Perfectly Normal</u> by Robie Harris is a great resource for boys and girls. Be sure you read it first.

As boys ask questions or make jokes, fill in the gaps. This is an age where there are some sexual innuendoes in their play and jokes. They think it is funny, but they are clueless as to why! I maintain that if we explain and take the "taboo"ness out of it, they cease the behaviors.

10. This is a good time to think about music. Music enhances the brain pathways for math and science. It increases their SAT scores, gives your children a skill to use all through life, and is a source of relaxation. It apparently increases the ability to get into medical school (and law school, I hear). Your child needs to take six months of lessons before he can pass judgment (by saying I hate this…). All music is BORING at first. (I still try and use the "I carried you for nine months" —talk about BORING! —routine"). It works sometimes and is always entertaining.

Go on field trips with your children at this age. They still want us. Say prayers. Tell them stories. Tell them how great they are. Point out their positive qualities and be specific. They are all too aware of their negative ones. Happiness comes in brief moments of connectedness. They enjoy fun stories about when they were babies. Do not compare two siblings, cousins, or anyone else (Why can't you be like so and so?). We are all individuals. My youngest has learned how to keep his mouth shut and work us to get what he wants. I know what he is doing. The oldest runs his mouth all the time and never gets anything. I told the older one to observe his brother's fine art of kissing up. He might want to try it. It is his choice. This way there is not true comparison but observation of behaviors that have positive outcomes, even if slightly manipulative.

Now share this next section with your child. I am going to tell him something very important! Your parents WANT to give you privileges. They want you to have everything possible. They love you. You must earn it. You earn it by doing whatever your parents ask THE FIRST TIME. You do whatever is asked of you without whining, complaining, or saying things like, "Why can't my sister (brother) do it? Why do I always have to? I did it yesterday. Brother (sister) never has to do anything…" Try not complaining and then do what your parents ask THE FIRST TIME for seven days. See how they change and what privileges you earn. I guarantee this works. It's up to you.

Ht_____   Wt_____

Eleven- to Thirteen-Year Visit
Middle School

Nostalgia: a key ingredient for this age. Pull out those baby pictures and remember how sweet your child was; how innocent, cooperative, full of potential he (she) was, and how everything you said was gospel. Remember how your child ran to you for hugs when he just needed one, or when he was hurt? Remember how he longed to be just like you and do everything with you? How you could fix anything? How powerful and magical you were?

This alien, who now inhabits your angel's body, needs to be removed. Exorcism seems like a good idea, as do boot camp and military school. What night was it when that sweet child went to bed and woke up possessed? When did you become the world's stupidest person? Why is it, that no matter what we utter, it is wrong? My kids challenge me on medical facts! I told my son to show me his medical degree, so he ran and made one!

In ancient tribal times, this is the age that boys were removed from their mothers, taken by their fathers to become men, and trained in the ways of the warrior. Knowing that helps me see my son as a savage who needs to be taken away and taught to be a man. It also helps me see through his behavior at times and understand that he is trying to be grown up, and trying to separate. He just doesn't know how. It is a struggle and a process. Daughters have permanent PMS and cry about everything. Mood swings make you think that Prozac for everyone might be beneficial! Now the real monkey wrench in all this is that our children need us more than ever. They need the steady boundaries and the guiding hand to help them grow. My son fussed one night when I was asking who he was talking to online and what were they talking about. He said, "Gee, Mom, other kids' parents are pulling away from their kids' social life. Why are you so interested in mine?" He has such a great way of identifying the exact reasons we do things! I told him he was lucky we are so interested.

It is essential, even life saving, that you stay one step ahead of your child at this point. You must remember that you are bigger, smarter, and have more knowledge. WE ARE THE ADULTS. We still make the rules and enforce them. Be inventive with consequences. Be creative with your words.

Explain the long-term consequences of certain behaviors. Remember when your child is blaming you for everything that has gone wrong since the BIG BANG, that whatever is wrong in his life ultimately resorted from his choice. It wasn't you who told him to say rude things or be sassy…that was his doing, all alone. You are simply happy to follow through with consequences. Tabasco still works at this age.

It wasn't you who decided to go to a friend's house and not tell anyone where you were, so your parents freaked and called the police. No, your child did that all by himself. It wasn't you who told your child to wait until the last minute to do a project that counts 50 percent of his grade. Certain choices have definite consequences! Let him learn. It is painful, but the more painful it is, the less likely he is to repeat (within reason…duh!). Keep in mind that the more you "rescue" him or her from bad choices, the more you reinforce unwanted behavior. Be clear on how and why you "rescue" your child.

Your middle schooler can definitely learn to do laundry—fluff, fold, and put it away. It is essential that boys throw their dirty socks, underwear, and workout "stuff" in the laundry or their room will smell like a locker room for days! In general, an adolescent needs to be fourteen years old to mow the lawn. It is not safe for kids to drive riding lawn mowers or ride on them. You must be sixteen to drive a car, truck, or van. It is still a must to wear helmets on their heads if they bike, rollerblade, scooter, or skateboard. (I see kids all the time with their helmets on their bicycle handlebars!) Contrary to popular opinion, adolescents do NOT know everything. The emergency rooms are full of bad accidents that resulted from bad choices—dangerous choices by people who thought they knew everything.

If you have not discussed puberty, do so! You do not want your children learning from friends who do not have all the facts. Discuss drugs, alcohol, and sex with them. Be clear on why these are bad choices. AIDS is not an adult-only disease. Tell them about "huffing," or sniffing, household chemicals. This is readily available-huffing can kill or at least ruin your child's life.

If they do not know the meaning of all those bad words they hear in school, tell them. Discuss bullying, bigotry, and prejudice. Tell them how racist jokes are not funny. They are exposed to so much. They need to know what is right and wrong and purely mean. Discuss the "sensuality" of puberty. This means the feelings they have, and their senses. Teach them to see both sides of an equation or conflict. <u>See things from the other person's point of view.</u> This is a great life lesson that can resolve conflicts. Physical aggression (the preferred method for boys) is not the answer to all conflict, nor is backstabbing (the preferred method for girls). <u>The Last Lecture</u> by Randy Pausch is a fantastic book with a lot of nice life lessons for our children.

When you think you have lost him or her totally, he will do or say something that makes you realize that he is listening. Keep at it. Teens are really like toddlers. They want to know you are there to catch them if they fall, but they want to strike out on their own as much as possible. We are there with enough rope to go just so far, and then we reel them in for safety. They want and need to know someone cares.

If your child has computer privileges, restrict his Internet access. He should not answer any e-mail with a name he does not know. She should not talk or e-mail anyone she does not know in the flesh. Know who your child's friends are. Be the keeper of her password. Know the games he plays. Limit his time on Internet games, as well as Nintendo, PS1, 2, 3, or XBox, etc.

Be clear on rules. Follow through on consequences. Keep firearms away from him—locked up and ammunition separate. Your child should know how to swim and know water safety if you are around water. No horseplay around the pool. Don't bounce balls in the house. Don't throw things in the house. Don't torture your sister (brother). Put your things away, etc.

Last but not least, I tell children all the time that we as parents really do want to give them privileges. They have to earn it by doing what we ask the first time. I challenge them to test this for a week.

Consciously do what is asked of you without back talk, excuses, etc, and watch the transformation in your parents. See what privileges come your way (within reason!). It is not difficult to raise parents. They need appreciation, and they need for you, the child, to do what you are asked. Simple. And the kids just don't get it!

Your child needs a tetanus booster shot at twelve, before entry into seventh grade.

Your child may also need a meningitis vaccine, the Menactra. Gardasil is also recommended for girls to prevent HPV (human papilloma virus). Currently, I am not recommending this vaccine, as it has had too many negative side effects. Perhaps in another two to three years it will be better. I also believe that your daughter should be included in a decision that directly affects her decision to become sexually active.

Ht_____Wt_____

The following books are recommended, and are fabulous!!!

1. Sean Covey, The 7 Habits of Highly Effective Teens
2. Wolfe, Get out of My Life, But Can You Drop Me and Cheryl at the Mall
3. Ruiz, The Four Agreements
4. Larson, All the Far Side books for Mom and Dad. (Sometimes you just need to laugh)
5. Chapman, The 5 Love Languages of TEENAGERS (this is a necessary book for all parents)
6. Nelsen, Jane, Positive Discipline for Teenagers
7. Randy Pausch, The Last Lecture

Fourteen-Year Well-Visit

This will be an expansion of the thirteen- to eighteen-year well-visit. When last we talked, we wondered from whence came the alien that occupied our child as he or she became a teenager. Well, it took me a year, but I figured it out. It came from his father. There is simply no way that I, the mother, had anything to do with the hideous transformation of my angel child into a teenage horror.

At fourteen, your child is either in eighth or ninth grade and totally pubertal or non-pubertal. Either way, it is no fun as a parent. If your child is a daughter, you so know the eye rolling and the exasperated sigh as if you have committed some mortal sin. If your child is a son, he no longer wants you to be a part of his life, except to cart him here and there, give him money, and approve of all he does and does not do. It is easier to pay someone to do extra work around the house than to get a teenager to do anything willingly or even pleasantly!

Yet, I know you see something there—a glimpse of hope that perhaps all is not lost. It comes at odd times. He or she will suddenly say, "I love you," or thank you for no apparent reason. Or you come home and find his room clean. Sorry, scratch the clean room. That is only my delusional thinking. Where did this child learn all those bad vocabulary words? I know I didn't know those bad words until I was in college. I would go talk to his teacher (not about the bad words, but about his academic performance) except that he told me I would "totally" ruin his life if I did.

Fourteen is an age that has baffled me for twenty years. What was God thinking when he made the fourteen-year-old? The fourteen year old is not a kid, and he or she is definitely not an adult. He or she does not think anything through, and at fourteen, most teens think they are invincible. It is the beginning of parental stupidity (we cannot understand anything!); and apparently none of us was ever a teenager.

I highly recommend the book Positive Discipline for Teenagers by Jane Nelsen, and I recommend you actually read it. On days that

I feel our ship is sunk, I stop and reflect on my teen. Sometimes you have to look at what they have <u>not</u> done, as well as what they have done. As parents, we know where our teens are. We know their grades. We know they tell us when they're not doing well in school, before we get the progress reports. We know their interests, their friends, and their feelings about drugs and alcohol.

The process of growing up and separating from one's child(ren) is difficult. It is crucial to lay out the ground rules. Be sure you as a parent follow them as well, specifically on dating, driving, drinking, doing drugs, and having sex without planning. Let your child know what will happen when he or she does poorly on the report cards.

Find time to just be—without talking (which is EXTREMELY hard for me as I love to talk and share feelings). Play noncompetitive board games (Let me recommend Chicken Soup for the Soul board game). Ask specific questions about their friends and their school. Sometimes we should lecture, and sometimes we should keep our mouths shut, as talking too much drives them away. When sharing significant "values" stories with your children, be sure it is simply a teaching tool and not an attempt to make them feel like you are judging them. You do not want your children to think they would behave in such a negative manner.

I also recommend watching the movie Freaky Friday (the one with Jamie Lee Curtis). It is really a cute movie, and it made me stop and think how I would fare if I were transposed into my child's body. I realized I would not fare well. It gave me new respect for my son's life.

As parents, we are still strict and have rules. We try to listen to our boys. My boys recently gave me specific examples that showed how little I really listen to them, and how much I tune them out. I have learned that they can teach me, when I choose to be aware.

I have learned from other parents that this is a phase, and it is best to hang in there, as children do improve. I only hope they improve while I still have memory cells left. I also hope to restructure my life so that I have more fun. My kids structure their lives so that (unfortunately) FUN is the priority. This is not all bad, as we adults have structured our lives so that FUN is not a priority—universal balance, people! So if I have more fun, he will study more. (Do not mess with my delusions. I am happy with them).

So fourteen becomes fifteen, and then you have a child who wants to drive. I have discovered that there is huge leverage with this desire. Since it involves responsibility and freedom, I can absolutely make the rules that will allow for this PRIVILEGE (yes, it is not a right, as they would have us think) to happen. I also have freely discussed the financial impact of this privilege, and it really can be up to your child to step up to the plate and take responsibility for his or her driving privilege. Decide if you will pay for gas and/or car insurance. Decide ahead of time what financial responsibility your child will have with driving. What happens if he or she gets a ticket? What will constitute having his license taken away, or the car?

Remember, there is light at the end of the tunnel. It is NOT an oncoming train. Rejoice in all that is good with your child. Remember it is more effective to discipline <u>without</u> anger. Write a contract if you need to. Now is a time when the self-confident, self-assured child that you have raised may indeed point out where you are role modeling poorly. Some parents may find this concept offensive. (I do if the discussion is presented poorly.) If my child points out a valid misbehavior of mine, I acknowledge it and make plans to improve. How can I expect him to change if I do not?

Well, good luck. The great thing is that there are plenty of parents with teens who are an automatic support group. As difficult as this time is, it is necessary for your child to become an independent, and not a co-dependent, adult. Find balance—your career, his life, fun for you, fun for him, and family time. Jane Nelsen said it best, "Become their co-pilot." You no longer need to pilot their plane, but we must keep them from going down in flames! It is a time to find your own hobby while still being around for your teen to lean on. Offer suggestions rather than tell them what to do. Ask them how they would solve a particular problem. They have skills you know nothing about—good skills!! Catch them doing something right.

HT_____ WT_____ BP_____

BOOKS:

1. <u>Raising a Son</u>/<u>Raising a Daughter</u> by Don and Jean Elium (these are two separate books)
2. <u>Get Out of My Life but Take Me and Sheryl to the Mall</u> by Wolfe
3. <u>Positive Discipline for Teenagers</u> by Jane Nelsen
4. <u>The Five Love Languages of Teenagers</u> by Campbell and Ross
5. <u>The Bible</u> (I have found that many kids like hearing their parents read aloud a little every day)
6. Eldredge, John, <u>Captivating</u>
7. Eldredge, John, <u>Wild at Heart</u>
8. Pausch, Randy <u>The Last Lecture</u>

Fifteen to Seventeen Years Old

Well, we made it to fifteen! I did not think we would survive fourteen, but we did, and now we hope this will be a better year.

Your teen is now in ninth or tenth grade. Wow, we feel so old because our baby is growing up so fast. Ninth grade is another big transition year, and if your child enters a large high school (like ours did with 3500 students in the school), it is important to set the rules of conduct for school. Expectations must be clear, as well as consequences. In a BIG school, your child can easily get lost in the social process, and forget he or she is there to get an education! Know his or her teachers. Our sons' teachers are more than willing to e-mail and keep us up to date. It really helps to know what is going on in their lives during the eight hours they are not with us.

The "magnet" (honors) programs in Orlando offer some real benefits if your child is so inclined. In these programs, your child has the same teachers for four years and is in class with the same students. It gives the "small school feeling" in a big city environment. It takes a very special person to do the IB (International Baccalaureate) programs, as those are really academically accelerated, and the kids do not have much time for anything else. I do not care for these programs at this time, and for that reason. I think high schoolers need to have a balance of work and play. We all do!

It is also important for your high school child to have some extracurricular activity—some sport or regular involvement in a club or parent-approved activity. Those teens left to their own devices tend to get in trouble.

As parents, we also make a point of knowing who are sons' friends are. We are strict about who they ride with and where they are going. We require they be home at identified times, and we do not tolerate being late. We have discovered that holding our children accountable for their actions is very important, and we do not let them bend the rules. Our kids are very bright, and when they can get an inch, they take a mile.

Now that your teen is fifteen, let's talk about driving.

It is important that as parents, you decide when and under what circumstances your child can get a permit to drive. Some parents think grades are important, behaviors, etc. I used to. Then I realized that my child needs the experience while we have control, and the longer he can drive with a permit, the better off he will be. Having a permit allows the child to drive with someone age twenty-one and over. Your "permit" driver does not have to be added to the insurance policy. The child cannot get a driver's license until (minimum) one year after getting the permit, and with parental permission! We required our children at fifteen to get permits so they had a longer time to obtain experience. I cringe at the idea of their being eighteen and being able to drive with little to no experience. I also encourage driver's education with "real time" driving. A lot of high school programs use simulators. My kids have been doing that with video games for a long time. I needed to have "real life" behind the wheel training with a real person. The Florida Safety Council provides a great course, and it's worth every penny.

As parents, we also require a B average to drive, as our insurance rates are decreased with a B average. Our policy is reduced $426.00 every six months ($952.00 a year) if our teen driver has taken driver's education and has a B average. That is a lot of savings!

I hope your teen fulfills your dreams for him or her. Ours have not. We have had to step back and look at the big picture. A lot of the time what we want them to be, and what God wants them to be, are two different things. We are clear that life-altering or life-threatening behaviors are not tolerated—drinking, drugs, lying, stealing, skipping school, etc. We have to individualize other issues. We wanted them to go to a four-year college. We wanted them to have all As and Bs. We wanted them to be excellent students. Well, they didn't have all As and Bs, and the reality is they may have to go to community college initially. Or they may have to take a year off, learn about the real world, and minimum wage jobs initially. NOT what we would pick, but if this is the best way for them to learn, then so be it. It is better to work with them than against them. We often stop and think, "What do we really want?"

We want happy, successful children leading productive lives. There are a lot of ways to accomplish that. We want good communication and a healthy relationship, which cannot occur if there is always fighting. So, we co-pilot them rather than pilot them and control their every move. It is tough stepping into the co-pilot seat when you have been flying the plane all these years. We hold to the idea that we do not want them living with us at age forty! Our lives have been spent getting them to a point of independence and maturity. It just feels odd when it gets here. Empty nest is real, and it starts before they leave. It begins slowly as they become independent and spend more time with their friends and less with us. They are trying to find themselves, and we stay here guiding so they do not make really BAD choices. If they do make bad choices, we are here to help them change.

Journey with joy. I have found that even in conflict, I learn something and my children have helped me evolve. Why yes, I freely confess there are MANY days I do not like teenagers…anyone's! The magnitude of dislike is proportional to the amount of conflict I have at home, but then it passes. When there is a really good day, you can see that all is not lost, and you are not the worst parent on the planet!

We connect with other parents, too. There is great fun in commiserating with other parents, as all teens seem to be alike— "support groups," as it were. Comparing notes helps keep the perspective that you are doing a good job, and that your kids are really good kids underneath all the rebellion. Continue to catch them doing something right. Hearing that you have done something nice or done something well goes a long way. Use your sense of humor. I tell my boys they drive me crazy, and these days it is a short trip. We have a list of "things you thought you would never say," such as, "Yes, son, you can get your ears pierced. Wow, you brought your grade up to a 62! I am so proud of you (it was a 31). Yes, you can drive to the beach today. How do we guarantee that he will fail this semester?" So life is full of funny and fun moments. Make the most of them. Those are the moments that keep you sane and remind you why you had children in the first place.

*Ht*_____ *Wt*_____ *BP*_____

Eighteen Years Old

Ah! At last, almost Nirvana. Something marvelous happened at eighteen (for us). As surely as he was possessed by demons at an earlier age, our son became un-possessed. It happened a month after graduation. We were so concerned he would not graduate because he had missed so many days in high school. Nevertheless, he DID graduate and was accepted to college. He had no specific focus at that time, but a month later, he came home with direction and goals.

Suddenly (really) we had a common ground and could talk about adult things. He announced he wanted to go into the medical field (yes, it actually was a surprise), and now we could relate to him in complete thoughts and sentences.

He got a job and went to college. The light at the end of the tunnel was in fact, NOT an oncoming train, as we had feared. He has chosen to live at home the first year to get grounded and adjusted to college life expectations. Then he will move out. (He moved out after the first semester. At the end of his first year in college, he realized it was not for him, and he joined the Marines. We've never seen him happier nor have we been more proud. This was quite the curve ball but has worked out well).

So, as many parents had told me in practice, you must wait them out. MOST teenagers do come around. There are always the few who spoil everything, but most find their children do return to sanity and become productive citizens.

Stick to your rules and values. Do not budge on the important matters in your home. Offer advice, knowing he or she will not accept it. Take heart and know that your children do listen and incorporate it when you least expect it.

We did tell our son that one of the many reasons to go to college is health insurance. If your eighteen-year-old is not in school and is working, then your health insurance will drop him or her without your consent. Some car insurances will do the same. Your eighteen-year-old is an adult, and if working, is responsible for him or herself. Because of HIPAA changes, your adult child has to make medical decisions for him or herself. The college your child attends will not tell you his or her grades without prior written consent from the child. Even though you pay for the education, the child is accountable and responsible for his or her own grades.

Your eighteen-year-old is technically an adult, but still very much a child needing guidance. Enjoy the transition. It is truly amazing.

Ht_____WT_____ BP_____

Dreams:_____

1. Young, William, <u>The Shack</u>
2. Pausch, Randy <u>The Last Lecture</u>
3. Chapman, <u>The Five Love Languages of Teenagers</u>
4. Meyer, Joyce <u>Conflict Free Living (a very spiritual book)</u>

Chapter Three
What To Do When
Your Child is Sick

Asthma

Asthma is a condition that involves inflammation and constriction of the airways. It has an underlying allergic predisposition and a high hereditary component. If one parent has allergies or asthma, the children have a 30 percent risk of developing it. If both parents have allergies and/or asthma, then there is a 60 percent probability the children may develop the same. If the mother has asthma, there is a high probability that the children may develop asthma by age six. (This is a new statistic that is interesting. Why age six? We do not know but statistics are showing this is what happens.) New studies also indicate that there is an increased risk of developing asthma by age seven if a child receives antibiotics in the first year of life.

Asthma is also becoming known as part of an "allergy march" where a person may initially just have allergies with runny nose, itchy eyes, etc. Over time, the illness progresses to eczema and then asthma.

There is no single test to predict who will get asthma so we cannot "prevent" a person from getting it.

However, there are steps that can be taken to minimize symptoms. If there is a family history of asthma/allergies, then trying to reduce the development of symptoms from birth is an ideal situation. Breast-feeding is the first line of defense, if possible. Breast-feeding for four months (minimum) helps reduce the incidence of lower respiratory infection during the first year of life. Such infections can precipitate asthma. If mom cannot breast-feed, then do not use a milk-based formula. If there is a family history of soy problems then a soy-based formula should probably not be used. Discuss with your doctor what formulas would be best under these circumstances.

Once foods are introduced, do not use cereals (grains can be sensitizing in predisposed individuals. There is usually little problem with rice cereal); go straight to vegetables and fruits, and introduce one *new* food every five to seven days. Do not introduce foods until after four months of age. By introducing foods slowly, a parent can determine if there are some delayed sensitivities. (Milk is the biggest allergen around. Delayed reaction to milk-based products can manifest as eczema, congestion that does not seem to go away, chronic loose stools, or even constipation. It does not appear immediately but after a few days to even weeks. It pays to be alert to what your child is eating, and make a note about anything that occurs out of the ordinary.) I recommend skipping cereal that contains gluten. Gluten can be a sensitizing food and it is found in oatmeal and cream of wheat. Whole grain rice or rice cereal (from Earth's Best) is okay, but there is no real medical need when veggies and fruits are better. These strategies can enhance the immune system and decrease the potential for allergies to develop. New studies indicate the ideal time to introduce foods is between four and six months of age. There is apparently increased risk for food allergies to develop if food is introduced before four months and a slightly increased risk when food is introduced after six months. (see four month visit for details on foods).

Probiotics can also help by keeping the intestinal balance of bacteria. (Infants need Bifidus Bifidobacterium: dose is 1/8 tsp 2x a day in infancy and after four months up to ½ tsp 2x is fine.) Mom can take fish oil or other omega three fatty acid supplements.

(Fish oil needs to be pharmaceutical grade. This means it has been processed to remove mercury. Please do not buy fish oil anywhere except reputable health food stores or online from reputable dealers. Expecta is an algae-based omega three fatty acid that can be found at Walgreen's, Target, and Albertsons.) When the child is over a year, the child can take omega three fatty acid supplements. Prior to that, it is best if Mom takes the omega three fatty acids and breast-feeds or the infant takes a formula enhanced with DHA (Most of them are these days).

Reducing allergy exposure in the house can help, too. It is important NOT to keep the house too clean as exposure to germs does help build immunity. Recent studies also show that having a furry pet or two in the home during the first year of life can help reduce the development of allergies. Also living on a farm—or visiting one frequently—has a beneficial affect on the immune system. Apparently, exposure to the fungi toxins and other farm germs boosts the immune system. These "ordinary" germs stimulate the healthy immune system. By living too germ-free, our immune system tends to develop more of the allergy antibody IgE. (Since nothing is 100 percent with people or medicine, there will be the one or two that this all backfires on. Those people's systems are just allergic!)

Having no carpet in the home helps. Tile or wood floors help reduce the dust and dust mites that live in the carpet and pads. Tile or wood is easier to clean. Keeping the mattresses and pillows in hypoallergenic coverings will also help.

If a child does develop allergies/asthma anyway, then the child needs treatment. The Franz Center offers traditional and alternative therapies for allergies, but NOT for asthma. "Breathing is fundamental!" When a child develops asthma, traditional medicines must be used so the child can breathe. Alternative therapies can be introduced in *non-crisis* times to help the immune system and prevent future occurrences.

MILD allergic symptoms can be helped with over-the-counter medicines like Claritin, Alavert, Benadryl, Dayquil, and Zyrtec. Nasal steroids are also very helpful by reducing swelling in the nose where allergens hit first. The medicine Singulair can be helpful as well.

Homeopathic Remedies for Acute Allergies

1. Allium Cepa (Homeopathic remedy made from the onion) can also alleviate symptoms of profuse clear drainage from the eyes or nose, like when you are cutting an onion.

2. Hydrastis Candidensis can help with yellow secretions, tickling in the nose, burning in the nose, and drainage that is worse in open air. When there is rawness of the nose, frontal headache, nosebleeds, this remedy can really help.

3 .Euphrasia is good when the eyes are red and tearing. There is profuse watery discharge from the eyes and nose. Generally, the patient feels better in open air. The margins of the eyelids may feel dry. There may be sensitivity to light as well.

These remedies can be tried to see if there is relief from the symptoms. Other testing can be done to help minimize symptoms. I use dried blood analysis, and this helps identify other system problems that may provoke allergy symptoms. There is no cure for allergies at this point.

Acute asthma is treated with traditional medicines. Studies show that people who treat asthma with alternative therapies *alone* do worse than patients who use traditional medicine alone or in combination with alternative therapies. Further research also shows that asthma is primarily a result of airway inflammation, which leads to the constriction that causes problems breathing.

Inhaled steroids are the primary treatment. They are safe and essential! Being on inhaled steroids for two years every day allows the lungs to remodel and improve function in patients with moderate to severe asthma. In addition, inhaled steroids do not interfere with growth and development.

Inhaled steroids taken <u>every day</u> for three years are equal to the same amount given orally for three days.

<u>While there are alternative therapies for asthma, they must be sought in conjunction with traditional medical care for the best outcome.</u> It is unfair and unwise to allow your child to have long-

term lung damage when suitable and proven therapy is available because you would prefer "natural medicine." Asthma is not a natural condition. Do what is necessary for you or your child to breathe; then seek other ways to improve health overall. As overall health improves, then the natural course is to see that medications can be weaned because they are no longer needed.

Colic

Parents often ask about colic, and I tell them do not ask unless their child has colic because it is a parent's nightmare—a beautiful new baby who screams 24/7 and is only quiet during feeds.

We don't know the exact cause for colic. There are two general theories, and I can only remember the one that I believe in—that the digestive system is too immature to digest properly. The inability to properly digest food/milk leads to colicky pain. Perhaps some abnormal protein absorption leads to abnormal peptide formation and abnormal neurotransmitters that cause irritation of the central nervous system.

The good news is that your child will outgrow this by four to six months of age (even if you do nothing). In the meantime, the hardest part is dealing with the constant crying and being patient. It is VERY difficult. There are several interventions that you can try that will ease the transition while we wait for the digestive system to mature. For some infants one of these therapies will be miraculous. For a very few, nothing will seem to work.

1. If your baby is exclusively breast-fed, mom should eliminate dairy from her diet, as it can be very irritating and allergenic in newborns. Dairy is the number one cause for food allergies. *Rarely* some moms will need to quit breast-feeding because it is the breast milk that is the problem, but this is rare. Stopping breast-feeding is not an option for discussion until all other avenues have been explored.

2. If your baby is formula-fed and colicky, then the first step is to go to a hydrolysate formula—one that is "predigested" so the infant's digestive system does little to no work on breaking down the nutrients needed to be absorbed. We recommend Alimentum or Nutramigen as first-line alternatives. These formulas are already broken down into their essential digestible and absorbable forms of nutrients.

3. We do not like to formula shop and try them all. I generally skip soy as the second step since 30-50 percent of kids who have a problem with dairy will have a problem with soy.

4. <u>Craniosacral therapy</u> is excellent in helping to prevent colic and in alleviating the tummy aches associated with it. It also helps resolve "birth trauma" and the abnormal head shapes that can result from long hard labor. It also enhances breast-feeding and latching on of the infant. It can be done anytime after birth and will definitely help alleviate (not cure) the symptoms of colic.

5. The number one *medical* recommendation is Mylicon drops. The simethicone helps break up gas bubbles. It is a bit expensive but a tried and true therapy. I tend to like the following therapies a bit better.

6. <u>Chamomile</u>—a homeopathic remedy that comes as little sugar pellets in doses marked 30c or 200c. This remedy is indicated and works well when "nothing seems to make the child happy, and the child is better if you walk and jostle" - constant "rough" motion. This is the child that you walk the floors with all night . . . literally. Homeopathic remedies are generally available at health food stores. Dissolve two pellets in water and give one dropper every two to four hours as needed. Homeopathic remedies are not drugs and do not have side effects. There is no magic

in dosing. It can be given numerous times a day for two weeks at a time.

7. Nux Vomica—30c or 200c—a homeopathic remedy. Dissolve two pellets in water and give one dropper as needed. This works well with an irritable baby that spits up. Actually both chamomile and nux vomica work for the irritable baby.

8. Cocyntal is one of the only combination remedies I like. It comes in liquid ampules that can be opened and used as needed.

9. Camilia—another liquid remedy that has had good success with many babies.

10. Lycopodium—30c is another good homeopathic remedy for the GI system. "Baby cries all day and sleeps all night."

11. Gripe water—a liquid that has been gaining in popularity over the last several years. Gripe water can contain any of the following ingredients:
    a. Anise to aid digestion
    b. Angelica to soothe upset stomach
    c. Caraway to relieve flatulence and indigestion
    d. Cardamom to relieves flatulence and indigestion
    e. Catnip to support digestion and relieve upset stomach
    f. Chamomile to settle the stomach
    g. Cinnamon bark to aid digestion and relieve flatulence and vomiting
    h. Dill to dispel flatulence, stimulate appetite, and settle stomach
    i. Fennel for stomach upset, hiccups, and gas
    j. Ginger to ease nausea and other digestive problems
    k. Sodium bicarbonate (baking soda) to decrease stomach acidity

12. Probiotics are "good bacteria." Many infants do not have the proper colonization of beneficial bacteria

in their intestines. Colic symptoms can be improved in these children by giving them the needed good bacteria by mouth. Bifidus Bifidobacterium is what is needed: one eighth tsp 2x a day in a newborn; ¼ tsp 2x infants 2-4 months; and ½ tsp 2x a day there after. One mother of eight has given this to all eight of her children as infants, and not one has had colic. Dissolve the powder in water and give to the baby by bottle or by dropper. It can be added directly to formula in the bottle-fed infant. While this is listed #12, it should be tried first! Studies in premature infants are showing that probiotic use decreases the incidence of developing a bad gut infection that premies are prone to get: NEC or necrotizing enterocolitis. If it helps with this bad infection, it should work wonders for colic!!!

13. Car Rides—an old remedy but one that should be included anyway. Riding in the car often appeases colicky infants. The constant motion and gentle hum seems to be positive. This is not a good idea when the parents are exhausted or the infant requires eight hours of riding to sleep. I tried to duplicate this by putting the baby in a safe basket on top of the dryer. The heat and rumble of the dryer should mimic the car ride. Not a good idea to leave the baby on the dryer unattended!

14. The last resort is a narcotic drop called Levsyn. The Hyoscyamine calms the digestive tract and knocks the baby out. There is a lot to be said for sleeping, but I do not use this unless all other options have failed. It is possible to get the baby addicted to this, but it can also be weaned. You can see why this is a LAST RESORT. Only a physician can prescribe it.

15. Before I entertain using Levsyn, I would like the baby to see a gastroenterologist—a GI specialist. Some of these babies need to have endoscopy where

they look at the intestines and see if there is a severe intestinal allergy. Many babies will have a milk protein enteropathy—a condition where the milk protein irritates the intestines and there is increased effort in digesting it. Fortunately, this is a temporary condition and they do outgrow it. The baby will need to be on a milk-free formula or breast-fed.

16. <u>Food allergies and digestive immaturity</u> seem to go hand in hand to create colic. Again, the good news is that all babies outgrow this with time. We continue to look for new and innovative ways to help it pass sooner as there is no cure because we do not know the cause. Perhaps probiotic use in all newborns would enhance digestion and prevent this all together!

Croup

Croup is a viral illness. It is typically caused by a parainfluenza virus and occasionally RSV, or Respiratory Syncytial Virus. It is a disease of the night with sudden onset between 10:00 p.m. and 4:00 a.m. The typical story is that parents put their well child to bed and around midnight he or she awakens "gasping" for air. The cough sounds like a seal or dog barking. Occasionally the sound of the cough is described as "sawing wood." The reason for the barking sound is that the tracheal (windpipe) mucous membrane becomes swollen, which narrows the airway. Air gets in fine but exhaling against a narrower exit makes the awful sound. On x-ray, the airway looks like a steeple or pencil.

Croup is scary but benign. It generally lasts one to three "bad" nights. A steamy shower is the first line of treatment and often offers relief. When that doesn't work, scared parents take their child to the emergency room. On the ride there, the air outside is cooler, and the child feels better, so by the time they arrive at the Emergency Department (ED), the child is better. Then it is okay to turn around and return home. Sometimes this is not so. In the ED, the treatment for croup is a single shot of Decadron (steroid). This steroid injection works wonders, decreasing the inflammation, offering symptom relief, and allows the body to finish the job of healing over the next couple days. A humidifier or vaporizer in the room may offer some relief as well. If you use a vaporizer, be sure no one can get burned on it.

Croup can occasionally be severe. While most cases are no worse than a common cold, there are indications that require medical intervention. Croup may also be treated with bronchodilators (Xoponex, Albuterol, Accuneb) to relax the airway, smooth muscles and decrease symptoms.

The following are symptoms that require evaluation in the emergency department:

- If the child has stridor—a high-pitched noisy inhalation (breathing in) or sounds like he or she is gasping for air with each inhalation.
- If the child begins drooling or has difficulty swallowing.
- If the child seems agitated or more irritable than normal. This can be a sign of hypoxia—low oxygen.
- If there is obvious struggling to breathe—the ribs are "sucking in" between the spaces or at the base of the throat.
- If the child becomes grayish or blue around the nose, mouth, or fingernails.

For uncomplicated croup, I recommend three homeopathic remedies that can make a big difference:

1. **Aconite**—30c or 200c at the onset of the illness. The onset is often missed and the remedy is not needed.
2. **Spongia**—200c. This remedy is the most commonly used for croup. Given at the start when you first hear the barky cough, it can make a big difference. Often after Spongia, the croup sound drops into the chest

and becomes a harsher more "chesty" cough. At this point, change the remedy to…

3. **Hepar Sulph** 30c or 200c. There is often a "ping pong" effect where the Hepar then makes the cough barky again. Repeat the Spongia. Then it is chesty again; repeat the Hepar. After that, it usually begins to get better.

4. Dissolve 2 pellets in enough water to give 1 ounce 3x a day for 2-3 days.

There are those special children who repeatedly get croup. A single daily dose of oral steroids (dosed at 2 mg /kg/day) at home can prevent a visit to the ED. This must be at the discretion of your physician.

Generally the child "croups" only for a night or two and the illness will finish like any other common cold. Often the child is better all day and croups only at night. In my experience, the child who croups all night and into the day will need steroids to decrease the inflammation. Otherwise, the second night is much worse than the first.

For those who cringe at the mention of steroids, remember that Breathing Is Fundamental! If your child cannot breathe and a little steroid fixes it, it is worth it!

Knowing what croup is, and what to do, helps keep you calm, which in turn keeps your child calm. Having the information to follow if symptoms increase also helps. As one of my favorite quotes goes, "And knowing is half the battle." That GI Joe doll knew so much in his day.

Diarrhea

Diarrhea is defined as excessive and frequent evacuation of watery feces, usually indicating gastrointestinal distress or disorder. It can develop as a result of a viral or bacterial infection. It may be the result of a toxin that irritates the intestinal cells and causes them to purge as a way of eliminating the threat. Parasites can cause diarrhea, as can food irritants or allergies.

Breast-fed infants have very loose yellow stools that are not considered diarrhea. Once children begin to have formed regular stools, parents know when there is a variation. The explosive, noisy, cramping, foul-smelling stool that often is diarrhea is difficult for even an inexperienced parent to miss!

Diarrhea is a healing response to an intestinal insult. The body wants to shed itself as quickly as possible of the offensive germ, and what better way than to literally flush it out. Sometimes the body is a bit too enthusiastic in its response or the offending agent is very malicious, and then there is rapid loss of fluid and weight, which results in dehydration.

Diarrhea with dehydration is still one of the leading causes of death in third-world countries. The body is roughly 85 percent water and when a person becomes dehydrated, an uncorrected dehydration leads to a total body shut down.

The treatment is simple—fluids, fluids, fluids—either orally or by intravenous route. Most diarrheic illnesses can be fixed with oral fluids. Children need fluids with electrolytes (salts and sugars) in them. Plain water dilutes the electrolytes in the blood and can lead to low sodium and then seizures. Children need Pedialyte, watered down Gatorade, chicken broth, ginger ale, etc. If the child has only diarrhea, he/she can actually be fed regular food, including milk. Studies have demonstrated effectively that with diarrhea alone, feeding through it is the best therapy. The stools will be bigger, but the nutrition speeds healing and the length of illness is reduced. Weight loss is reduced as well.

Dehydration is simple math. Intake must be more than output. If a child has had only eight to ten ounces of fluid intake and has had eight to ten watery stools, it is not difficult to realize that output was more than intake. Mild dehydration is a loss of 5 percent body weight. Severe dehydration is a loss of 10 percent body weight. Generally, severe dehydration requires IV fluids and often an overnight admission to correct the losses effectively.

If a child has two to five diarrheas a day and is drinking, medical intervention is unnecessary. The body has an appropriate response and the patient is able to keep up fluids, so we let it run its course.

Most mild diarrhea illnesses will run their course in three to five days. An increase above five stools a day or an increase in volume (the child has five **major** explosive stools a day…it goes everywhere!). Then we want to intervene and see if we can speed the healing process.

Fluids, fluids, fluids are still the number one therapy. Imodium AD can be used in the appropriate age group to SLOW the number of stools, and not stop them. If you stop them before the body is done, then the toxins percolate in the gut and there will be problems again.

I prefer well-selected homeopathic remedies for diarrhea. There are over 2,000 remedies available, and I wish to present a few that are commonly used with children, and tend to help most cases of diarrhea.

1. **Pulsatilla** is a great children's remedy in general. The child feels badly, is whiney, clingy, pitiful, and wants to be held all the time. The thirst is less than normal and the child may feel generally better outside. Symptoms tend to be a little worse around twilight (approximately 6:00 p.m.). When diarrhea occurs after a too-rich meal, this is the remedy—30c or 200c dissolved in water and given several times a day (two to five times) will improve symptoms.

2. **Arsenicum** (Yes, the remedy is made from Arsenic, but in homeopathic dilutions it is healing rather than toxic.) It is number one for food poisoning symptoms. When anyone gets acutely ill with vomiting and diarrhea, try Arsenicum first. It is also good for symptoms that are worse around midnight to 2:00 a.m. It is a good remedy if one has eaten bad meat or if one has burning pains (anywhere) that feel better with heat applied; 30c or 200c dissolved in water and given two to five times a day for two to three days maximum.

3. **Nux Vomica** is good for cramping pains that feel worse with pressure—nausea with the feeling that if

you could just vomit you would feel better. If one has the feeling that he/she has to go to the bathroom but cannot, nux vomica will resolve it. Stool can have mucous and/or blood mixed in it. Dosage: 30c or 200c dissolved in water and given two to five times a day for two to three days maximum.

4. Colocynthis is a great remedy for pain that "bends one double" or when one is curled up in a fetal position. Sometimes dairy is the reason for the pain and diarrhea, and Colocynthis will help. Dosage: 30c or 200c dissolved in water and given two to five times a day for two to three days maximum.

5. Podophyllum is excellent for diarrhea. Stools are often painless and explosive. It can be given with each stool and then the frequency decreases. You can use this remedy first and it will improve most cases of diarrhea. If it doesn't, then more details about the stools are needed. Dosing is the same as above: 30c or 200c dissolved in water and given two to five times a day for two to three days.

In traditional medicine, diarrhea is diarrhea. In homeopathy, diarrhea has a personality and the more observant you are, the more descriptive you are—then the better chance of finding a perfect remedy. Observe the color, intensity (explosive or not), smell (putrid, sweet, cadaveric—a great word meaning like a corpse), rotten egg, etc., chunky, watery, etc. What makes the child feel better (lying down, walking, sleeping, being carried, etc.)? When is it the worst (morning, evening, after eating, etc)? What makes the symptoms worse? All of these notations help a lot in choosing a remedy and helping the patient feel better.

As always, call your doctor if you are worried about your child. There is no substitute for an office visit. It helps the child, the patient, and the doctor. We cannot diagnose or properly assess a person over the phone. We can only offer general advice and hope it helps.

Eczema

Eczema is a skin condition of unknown etiology. We do not know the cause and believe it is genetic. We can treat it medically and keep it at bay, but there is no cure for eczema at this time.

A lot of eczema is related to food allergies, or at least some foods can worsen the symptoms. Milk/dairy is the biggest offender and the one food group to eliminate first. I also recommend doing allergy testing over one year of age, unless there is an infant with bad eczema and a family history of skin problems. Food allergy testing can be done via Immunocap for IgE testing or through labs like Sage or ALCAT. These latter two labs are generally not covered by insurance plans and their testing can run between $400.00 and $2,000.00.

For infants with a family history of allergies, asthma, or eczema, I recommend starting solids one at a time for seven days at a time rather than the usual three to four days at a time.

Medical treatment is primarily lotions (perfume free). Aquafor, Eucerin, Lubriderm, Crisco (butter free), castor oil, Olive oil, Calendula, or whatever lotion parents have found that works for their child. I put all kids on Omega three fatty acids as some mild cases respond miraculously to omega three fatty acids. It is like an internal emollient, and some people are deficient in omega three fatty acids. The most recommended omega three fatty acid supplement is cod liver oil.

Dosing is:
One to two years of age—one-half teaspoon a day
Ages two to five years—one teaspoon a day.

In our office we carry DHA Jr. Chewables. Coromega, which can be found at the health food store, is another good brand of cod liver oil. It is orange flavored cod liver oil in individual packets. I am a stickler about where you get cod liver oil, as it must be pharmaceutical grade and mercury free. Another good alternative is the algae based DHA in Expecta by Mead Johnson. These are gel caps and are not chewable.

A cream called <u>Schmoove</u> can also help with eczema. A Chinese herbal cream that is nutrition for the skin, it can be obtained in our office. We also carry a decoction (Chinese herbal tea) called Skin Tea (Restore Armor) that can help nourish the skin and improve eczema. This tea can help heal the eczema and prevent long-term problems.

Topical steroids are the medical mainstay for treating eczema. They suppress the inflammation and do improve symptoms, but they do not cure the problem. Once steroids are stopped, the eczema flares again. They are useful and indicated when there is a flare-up that really needs to be controlled.

Elidel is a topical non-steroidal cream that is also popular. It may cause some immunosuppression and is not a therapy I embrace. It also has its place for the severe eczema patient. Zyrtec, Claritin, and Atarax (hydroxyzine) may also help with severe itching at night.

It is important to notice if the child's eczema flares <u>after a</u> vaccination. (I am one of the few who believe that vaccines can aggravate eczema.) The use of homeopathic Silica 1M weekly times four to six weeks can help undo "bad effects" of a vaccination. Eczema aggravated at the seashore might respond to Carcinosin. Sulfur is another common remedy for eczema, especially if the eczema is worse while bathing, worse when scratching, better lying down, worse when sweating, hot, or red. Psorinum is a deep-acting homeopathic remedy for eczema, but not to be used lightly. These remedies should only be obtained from a homeopathic practitioner.

A recent article says breast-feeding (especially after a year) can contribute to a "leaky gut." I have had a couple children whose eczema improved once they quit breast-feeding and ate "regular" food.

Juice Plus™ Gummies are an excellent source of antioxidants and nutrients. They contain the whole food essence of seventeen fruits, vegetables and two grains in a gummy or pill form. (Need molars to eat these so will be best used in over eighteen-month-old children.) There are several antioxidant liquids as well. Mona Vie, Via Viente, Mangosteen, Noni Juice, and Pomegranate Juice are a few names of such products. Dermatology consults are often needed in the more challenging eczema cases.

More on Eczema

➤ Eczema is also called atopic dermatitis. It is one of the most common skin disorders in childhood and affects 17 percent of the childhood population.

➤ Onset during the first six months in 45 percent of children; first year of life in 60 percent of children. In 85 percent of affected children, onset is before five years old.

➤ Atopy comes from Greek word, *atopia* meaning "different" or "out of place." Atopic dermatitis is the more medically correct term.

➤ It is common to have asthma and allergic rhinitis at the same time.

Prevalence

➤ Twenty percent of the U.S. population has eczema. There has been a marked increase in the last several decades. In 1960, the prevalence was 3 percent.

➤ The increase in atopic dermatitis parallels the increase in asthma, which suggests shared triggers.

➤ Asthma occurs in up to 50 percent of children with AD (Atopic dermatitis).

➤ Allergic rhinitis develops in 50-85 percent of patients with AD.

➤ The more severe the dermatitis, the higher the risk of developing asthma as well as food sensitization and environmental allergies.

➤ AD occurs more often in urban than rural areas, and in higher socioeconomic classes.

➤ There is the belief that it stems from genetic alterations (There is a 75 percent concordance in monozygotic twins.)

➤ The condition will clear completely in 40-60 percent of patients at puberty or shortly after puberty.

Pathomechanism

Why eczema occurs is not really known or understood. There is a complex interaction between the immune system (immune dysregulation), the barrier protection of the skin (epidermal barrier dysfunction), and problems with medications (pharmacophysiologic abnormalities). The immune dysregulation explanation is too technical, and I will not elaborate on it. The abnormal barrier problem leads to increased loss of water from the epidermal layer and increased penetration of allergens, irritants and bacteria and/or viruses.

Clinical Features

> There is generally itching, redness, scaling, dryness, oozing, and bleeding. These problems can often be seen in the folds of the skin, the elbows, and behind the knees. The diaper may often be spared because it is warmer and wetter all the time and the diaper prevents penetration of microbes and irritants.

> There can also be plugging of follicles, called keratosis pilaris, circumoral (around the mouth) pallor, and irritation from saliva and foods. There is a commonly post-inflammatory hypopigmentation; decrease in pigment color of the skin which does resolve after six-plus months. We can also see Atopic pleats or lines under the lower lids. Palmer creases may be deeper as well.

> There is also a mild increase in molluscum contagiosum in atopic patients.

Infectious Complications

> Secondary infection is most commonly from *Staph aureus,* and occasionally *Strep pyogenes*. Bactroban (mupirocin) or the new Altabax can really help treat this superficial infection, as does oral Keflex (cephalexin).

➢ Eczema herpeticum is an explosive infection from HSV1 (Herpes Simplex Virus Type 1) and needs to be treated with acyclovir (an anti-herpes medicine).

Differential Diagnosis
➢ Seborrheic dermatitis
➢ Contact dermatitis
➢ Primary irritant dermatitis (saliva)
➢ Allergic contact dermatitis
➢ Nummular dermatitis (coin-shaped lesions or round plaques, commonly seen more in winter)
➢ Psoriasis
➢ Scabies
➢ Acrodermatitis enteropathica (which occurs from a zinc deficiency)

Family Impact
➢ Reduced quality of life, especially in those with moderate to severe disease.
➢ Reduced sleep due to itching and restlessness.
➢ Fatigue at school and limitation of sports participation.
➢ Increased fearfulness and dependence.
➢ Missed parent days from work and increased parental stress.

Management Medically
1. Daily baths, not greater than ten minutes, help hydrate the skin. The baths help remove surface bacteria and cause superficial desquamation of the skin.
2. Use of thick emollients after the bath increases skin moisturizing. It is best to apply them within three minutes after bathing. Aquafor, Eucerin, Lubriderm, Crisco (butter free), castor oil, olive oil, and Calendula are examples.
3. Use of mild soaps like Dove or Basis.

4. Adding Epsom salts to the bath can help detoxify the body and reduce stinging and itching.
5. Dressing the child in moist pajamas and socks that cling to the skin, topped by a dry layer to prevent excessive cooling; can be soothing and promote sleep.
6. Hydroxyzine can also help the child sleep. Hydroxyzine and Benadryl (equal parts) can work better together than either alone. Your healthcare provider must prescribe Hydroxyzine.
7. There is an old saying in dermatology, "If it is wet, dry it, and if it is dry, wet it."
8. With weeping oozing lesions, Burrow's solution (aluminum acetate) is germicidal and suppresses the weeping and oozing of acutely inflamed lesions. Apply two to three times a day for ten, fifteen-minute increments at a time with a *soft cloth*. Do this for up to five days. Washcloths are too heavy.
9. Avoid irritants and triggers. Overdressing children and inducing perspiration can irritate the AD. Swimming is excellent if the chlorine does not irritate the child. Sunscreen followed by a thick emollient before swimming can help protect from the chlorine.
10. Putting an emollient around the lips before eating can reduce the irritation of saliva and food with meals.
11. Soft cotton clothing reduces scratching and irritation.
12. Avoid use of harsh soaps, detergents, fabric softeners, and products with fragrance, and bubble baths.
13. Smoking around AD kids can increase the risk of asthma and irritate eczema.
14. Topical steroids and Elidel, which is prescribed by your healthcare provider.
15. Low concentration of bleach (1/4 to 1/8 cup) in a full tub can reduce secondary bacterial skin infection.

16. Bactroban in the nose two times per day for three weeks can reduce nasal colonization. Bactroban has a new "cousin," Altabax, which may be used on the skin for any irritated or infected lesions.
17. Children with eczema should not receive a smallpox vaccination or be around anyone who has recently had a smallpox vaccination.
18. Children with eczema should receive a chicken pox (Varivax) vaccination.
19. Schmoove topically –obtained from us or a licensed acupuncture practitioner in your area.
20. Skin Tea orally- obtained from us or a licensed acupuncture practitioner in your area.

Triggering Allergens

➤ Selective allergy testing (Immunocap) can help determine what the child is allergic to—environmental trees, grasses, dust mites, and a limited panel of foods.
➤ Food allergens are COMMON. At six months, 83 percent of patients with severe dermatitis show IgE food sensitization to milk, eggs, and peanuts.
➤ Sixty-five percent of these kids retain food sensitivity by twelve months old. (Five percent of six-month-olds and 11 percent of twelve-month-olds without AD show food sensitivities.) Citrus, wheat, milk, eggs, nuts, and soy are particularly aggravating.
➤ After the first few years of life, food sensitivity decreases but environmental (aeroallergens) sensitivity increases—dust mites, grasses, pollens, animal dander, and molds (particularly *Alternaria).*
➤ Allergen avoidance measures the following:
  1. Encasing mattresses and pillows
  2. Washing bedding in hot water weekly
  3. Vacuuming living areas frequently
  4. No stuffed animals

5. No carpet and no pets
6. All helps to decrease dust mite allergens and severity of dermatitis.
➢ Immunotherapy (allergy shots) is not as helpful with AD as it is with asthma and allergic rhinitis.

Alternative Medicine Approaches

1. Probiotics, especially Culturelle or Lactobacillus GG or *L. reuteri* can help reduce AD severity.
2. Probiotics can also reduce fungal overgrowth in the intestines, as there is some speculation that fungal overgrowth can worsen eczema.
3. Vaccines should be administered no more than one or two at a time. There are no studies or evidence that shots cause eczema, but I have seen eczema flare badly after vaccines.
4. Chinese herbal therapy. Schmoove "nutrition for the skin" and Skin Tea can decrease symptoms in conjunction with other therapies. This is available through practitioners only.
5. Arbonne skin products. (www.arbonne.com)
6. Epsom salt baths one to two times a week. Some patients' eczema responds well to salt water. Epsom salts can mimic the ocean as well as pull toxins out of the body.
7. Homeopathic Silica 1M weekly times four to six weeks can help undo bad effects of a vaccination. Eczema aggravated at the seashore might respond to the homeopathic remedy, Carcinosin. Homeopathic Sulfur is a common remedy for eczema, especially if it is worse while bathing, worse while scratching, better lying down, worse while sweating, and the rash is hot, and red. Psorinum is the ultimate remedy for eczema, but it is not to be used lightly. These remedies must be obtained through a trained homeopathic practitioner.

8. Omega three fatty acid supplementation—fish oil, Udo oil, total EFA. Expecta, etc., also helps improve eczema in many children.

9. An antifungal diet as well as antifungal creams may help in some cases.

10. Dried blood analysis.

11. Colostrum, derived from bovine colostrum, is dried and contains no dairy. It is rich in antibodies and growth factors that help heal the gut.

12. Stool testing through Genova Diagnostics can help determine if there is intestinal inflammation and the proper balance of intestinal bacteria.

13. Halleluiah Diet.

14. Eczemol, through Plymouth Pharmaceuticals, is a combination homeopathic remedy that claims to have benefits for eczema. Check this web site: www. plymouthpharmaceuticals.com.

15. Glyconutrients may also help as they are nutrition for every cell in the body. Check out www.Naturesunshine.com and www. GlycoDocs.org .

16. Cell Food with Silica is another product that may help, as it nourishes cells.

Febrile Seizures

Febrile Seizures are seizures that occur with a high fever. Febrile seizures usually occur between the ages of six months and two years of age. They can linger until age four or five, and most children outgrow them by age five years.

A fever is defined as a temperature greater than or equal to 101 degrees. A temperature is merely a measure of degrees, and everyone has a temperature. Even dead people have a temperature. An elevated temp over 101degrees is called a fever.

No one can predict who will or will not have seizures with fever, until they have one. If one of the child's parents had febrile seizures as a child, it is more likely their children will be predisposed to them, but not absolutely.

In my experience, most children who experience seizures with fever have a rapid rise in temperature over a short time span. Usually the fever is 102 and up, but I have seen children have seizures with a fever at 101-102 degrees. Fever, in general, is not a bad thing. Febrile Seizures are not a bad thing, either, but they are rather disturbing to watch. Fever is a result of the body's central thermostat responding to an insult, usually from a viral or bacterial infection. The brain's temperature controlling area, hypothalamus, raises the body's temperature (like turning on an oven) to cook the germ out. Some people's "ovens" are hotter than others. Some like to bake at 101 and some instantly go to broil at 104-105. We recommend letting a child remain at 101-102, as there is no harm in this degree of heat, and it can help the body defend itself. However, once a child has had a febrile seizure, this philosophy no longer applies, and an aggressive fever control becomes the norm. After a febrile seizure, we recommend acetaminophen and/or ibuprofen at the first sign of fever to keep it from elevating rapidly and potentially triggering a seizure.

Febrile seizures generally last less than five minutes (usually only one to two minutes). At the five-minute mark, call 911. There is nothing you need to do except time it. We no longer recommend putting a spoon in the mouth because patients do not swallow their tongues, and you can lose a finger that way. Just be sure the child is not in a dangerous spot where he can fall or hurt himself during the seizure. Place the child on a protected surface on his or her side. It is important to know how long the seizure lasts because it feels like an hour while it is happening. Timing it gives the parent something to do. After it is over, the patient is usually sleepy but returns to normal very quickly. With the first seizure, the child does need to be evaluated. Usually this evaluation will occur in an Emergency Department. Serious illnesses that cause fever must be ruled out. Once the diagnosis is established, the child does not need to go to the Emergency Department for every fever or every febrile seizure. Generally, further evaluation can be done in the pediatrician's office.

Children rarely have their first febrile seizure before six months or after three years. If the first seizure occurs under fifteen months of age, there is a statistically higher probability that the child may have them again. The older the child is at the onset of the first seizure, the less likely he is to have another one. One in twenty-five children will have a febrile seizure.

We do not know why some people have a lower threshold for seizures than others do. It is important to know that febrile seizures alone do not cause brain damage. Only one patient in one hundred will develop epilepsy after febrile seizures. Patients at higher risk for epilepsy after febrile seizures include those with a prolonged episode; greater than ten to fifteen minutes, those who have a seizure that involves only a part of the body, those who have a recurrence in twenty-four hours, and children with neurological problems.

Influenza, adenovirus, and parainfluenza are the three most common viral infections associated with febrile seizures in children.

Anticonvulsant therapy is rarely needed for simple febrile seizures, even if the child has a few of them. Medication is generally needed if there is a change in the pattern, or an increase in frequency and/or intensity.

Aggressive fever control is the medical management, as well as treating the underlying reason for the fever. The one extra treatment I recommend is homeopathic Belladonna in a potency of 200c. This can be given with each fever or even prophylactically in those who have had a few febrile seizures. Belladonna as a homeopathic remedy has its "keynote" or hallmark use when symptoms are "sudden onset, red, hot, and throbbing." A febrile seizure fits this description well. The rapid rise in temperature is the sudden onset, and fevers make us flushed (red), hot, and often there is throbbing or pulsing pain.

Strep Throat often presents acutely as well—red, hot, and throbbing. Strep often begins with a "little" sore throat and a few hours later the patient feels like a truck hit him and backed up for round two. The throat can be very red, and it hurts to swallow anything. **Belladonna** will also work wonders for this symptom picture. The remedy **Mercurius Vivus** works well when the throat hurts so badly the patient cannot swallow anything, including their own spit. <u>Medically, if a patient has strep throat, they also need to have a strep test done by the doctor's office and receive antibiotic therapy in addition to taking homeopathic remedies.</u>

Some strains of strep throat are "rheumatogenic," meaning they can cause rheumatic fever. It is unwise to refuse medical or antibiotic therapy for this condition. <u>There is no sense</u> in developing a deeper and more debilitating illness when penicillin, or its correct substitute for those who are penicillin allergic, works. I am all for homeopathic treatment and other alternative therapies when appropriate, but there are some illnesses that still need antibiotics! There truly are some risks that are not worth taking.

There are several great books on homeopathy for beginners. I am not here to reinvent the wheel or homeopathy. I wish to offer simple solutions that work in repeated situations. For more information, I recommend three beginner books:

1. Homeopathy at Home by M. Panos
2. Everybody's Guide to Homeopathic Medicine by D. Ullman and S. Cummings
3. Homeopathy from A to Z by D. Ullman

Head Injury

Head injuries are generally classified as open or closed.

Closed head injuries are more common and can be as minor as a bump or scrape on the head to as serious as coma, intracranial bleeding, and death.

Open head injuries always need evaluation in the emergency department.

This discussion is about minor closed head injuries and how to assess and manage them. Most children will fall and bump their heads at some point during childhood. It is simply a matter of how far and how fast they fell that help determines how serious the result of that incident is.

Accidents still account for the majority of deaths in children under five. Seventy-five percent of children under the age of one year will fall from a height of three feet or less before their first birthday. This is the height of a changing table, bed, kitchen counter, or chair. Most will result in minor injury. Many will get a concussion because of this fall. A concussion is merely a fancy medical word for a head injury. The severity of a concussion is graded as one through five. One is mild and five is a coma. A concussion means the brain was shaken inside the cranium.

When a child falls, the head, as it hits the ground, often makes that awful coconut sound. The head is fortunately very difficult to break, much like a coconut. The following is a series of questions and advice we give concerning head injury.

1. Did the child lose consciousness? If there is even a brief period of unconsciousness, the child needs to be evaluated in the emergency department (ED) right away. We are always concerned that a substantial fall will result in a bleed inside the head, and there is an increased risk of a bleed if there is a loss of consciousness. Such an injury requires immediate evaluation and intervention.

2. Did the child cry right away? Good. A fall is a scary thing and a child will usually cry afterwards because it scares him or her. This is an appropriate neurological response.

3. If the child is sleepy, let him or her fall asleep. It is impossible to keep the child awake, so do not try. More importantly, try to arouse them from sleep after about fifteen minutes. You should be able to elicit a response even if the child pushes you away and wants you to leave him or her alone. If you cannot rouse the child at all, then the child needs to go to the emergency department.

4. With concussions, the child will often vomit and turn pale. One time, maybe two is not alarming,

but if the child begins to vomit "like the exorcist" then the child needs to be seen in the emergency department.

5. A sudden decline in behavior with increasing irritability, belligerence, and/or combativeness also signals a problem and requires immediate evaluation in the emergency department.

6. The most significant problem is a bleed in the head, and will give some sign in the first twelve to twenty-four hours—loss of consciousness, change in behavior or level of consciousness, protracted vomiting, combativeness, or inability to awaken your child.

7. If the child fell from a height of six feet or more, he needs to be seen right away.

8. Most of the time the scenario is as follows: A child falls off a chair, out of a high chair, off the bed or changing table. It startles him or her. He cries immediately and scares everyone. He may be a little sleepy and may get a big goose egg on the head or he may throw up once. Then thirty minutes later the child is acting normal and as if nothing ever happened. This is not something you have to worry about. Once the child goes to bed, then try to arouse him or her from sleep (not fully awake, just enough to know they can be roused from sleep) every hour for two hours. Then relax and go back to your bed. If you cannot arouse him or her, a trip to the emergency department is in order.

9. Sometimes with a mild concussion, the child can experience headaches for a week to a month. In older kids, the headaches can sometimes be worse several days later, and the child may need some outpatient IV fluids. All this is not alarming.

10. Homeopathic **Arnica** in the potency of 30c or 200c can be given three times a day for three to four days,

which can also help. For children who have molars, the pellets can be chewed. For smaller children, dissolve the remedy in water and give about an ounce three times a day. This generally can be found at any good health food store (GNC is not a health food store).

11. Craniosacral therapy can help relieve, and even prevent, any headaches after a fall.

12. If you have any concerns, have your child seen by a physician. I have had good recovery from head injuries with concussions using Arnica. Sometimes I have to use a second remedy, Natrum Sulphuricum, which is indicated in a head injury with secondary problems. This should be obtained from a homeopathic practitioner.

Influenza

Flu is universal and occurs yearly. Every year the very young, the very old, and the immunocompromised are at highest risk for severe illness and death. Thirty-six thousand people a year die from this disease.

All flu viruses have their origins in birds. It has found a way to mutate and jump to humans from time to time, and then it can wreak havoc. Flu virus has a core with little spikes around it. The spikes are *neuraminidase* spikes and *haemagglutinin* spikes. Hence, you will see flu strains referred to as H1N1 or whatever number indicates the new strain. In 2007 the strain was H5N1 (**H**=haemagglutinin and **N**=neuraminidase). Each year's vaccine is generally based on last year's virus. The vaccines are made from killed virus. There is a new nasal vaccine for patients aged five to forty-nine that is a live virus (Flu Mist). The intent is to provide immunity and hope there is cross reactivity so that those vaccinated will not get so sick. The flu vaccine has been consistently proven to be 85 percent effective.

Until 2006, the flu vaccine for anyone over three years old contained the full dose of Thimerasol (25 mcg per dose). This amount of mercury per dose is cumulative in the body and has been the reason I have problems recommending the flu shot. I can more readily recommend the vaccine, now that it is mercury-free, for those who really need it or those who really want it.

As your physician, I can share my opinion about this vaccine. It is my policy to provide you with information and let you decide if this vaccine is right for you and your family. This practice usually has a limited supply and when it is gone, we generally do not get additional doses. During flu season, it is important to wash your hands, do your best to avoid being coughed or sneezed on, get plenty of rest, stay hydrated, and keep your immune system up.

Elderberry is the only herb proven to fight the flu, as it coats the little "N" spikes and prevents replication. Oscillococcinum is also available, and this homeopathic remedy can be taken prophylactically during high infection times and can be taken to treat symptoms early on as well. We carry **Allergy-Immune-Respiratory Tea** a Chinese herbal tea that works wonders on any respiratory mucous membrane affliction. Homeopathic remedies that may be indicated for the flu based on symptoms are Arsenicum, Bryonia, Gelsemium, Rhus Toxicodendron, and Eupatorium Perforatum. Again, you need to consult with a homeopathic practitioner if you cannot find simple symptoms in a good homeopathic book. *Homeopathy at Home* by M. Panos, or Ullman and Cummings' book, *Everybody's Guide to Homeopathic Medicine* can be great resources for simple infections that can be treated at home.

From the reading I have done, it seems the worst cases in 1918 were in those who took aspirin, which we now know causes Reye's syndrome when given during the flu or chicken pox infections. There were huge problems with overcrowding as WW1 was in full bloom. The crowded military camps enhanced the spread of the virus. It was a particularly virulent virus whose infectious ability became worsened by the crowding conditions and travel due to the war.

The media also over dramatizes EVERYTHING, so be cautious how much you watch, as the news will raise your anxiety level and hence decrease your immune level. I do not advocate being foolish, but I think there are enough sensible alternatives that being terrified of something that has not happened yet is unnecessary. It is true that the worst cases of flu cause respiratory problems and there are fatal cases. Most any illness can be rather benign or can be fatal in compromised hosts. The shot itself can cause illness and problems in susceptible patients.

Those with asthma, diabetes, cystic fibrosis, emphysema, or any chronic debilitating illness DO need to receive the vaccine yearly.

The following is extracted from the CDC influenza website:

"Influenza A virus is essentially an avian virus that has "recently" crossed into mammals. Birds have the greatest number and range of influenza strains. Avian haemagglutinin sometimes appear in pig human and horse influenza strains.

Every now and then (ten to fifteen years) a major new pandemic strain appears in man, with a totally new HA and sometimes a new NA as well (antigenic shift). This variant causes a major epidemic around the world (pandemic).

Over the subsequent years, this strain undergoes minor changes (antigenic drift) every two to three years, probably driven by selective antibody pressure in the populations of humans infected.

See the chart below indicating main pandemic strains in previous years.

Influenza A Evolution

1874—(H3N8)	
1890—(H2N2)	Pandemic
1902—(H3N2)	
1918—(H1N1)	Pandemic
1933—(H1N1)	First strains isolated
1947—(H1N1)	Variation detected

1957—(H2N2)	"Asian" Flu pandemic
1968—(H3N2)	"Hong Kong" Flu pandemic
1976—(H1N1)	"Swine" Flu, non-epidemic
1977—(H1N1) + (H3N2)	"Russian" Flu epidemic

This constant antigenic change through the years means that new vaccines have to be made on a regular basis.

New influenza strains spread rapidly in children in schools and in places where people crowd together. Influenza epidemics may cause economically significant absenteeism.

Influenza is characterized by fever, myalgia (muscle aches), headache and pharyngitis. In addition, there may be a cough and in severe cases, prostration. There is usually no coryza (runny nose), which characterizes common cold infections.

Infection may be very mild, even asymptomatic, moderate or very severe.

Source
The reservoir is acute infection in other human beings.

Spread
Aerial droplets and fomites rapidly spread flu, with inhalation into the pharynx or lower respiratory tract.

Incubation
Short duration, usually one to three days. Rapid spread leads to epidemics.

Complications
Tends to occur in the young, elderly, and persons with chronic cardio-pulmonary diseases.

Complications include:
1. Pneumonia caused by influenza itself.
2. Pneumonia caused by bacteria
   Haemophilus influenza
   Staphylococcus aureus

Streptococcus pneumonia
3. Other viral superinfection, e.g. Adenovirus.

Overall death rates increase in times of influenza epidemics."

Insect Bites

You have reached the most interesting part of this book. In fact, this information is worth the price of the book alone! Children get lots of insect bites—fleas, mosquitoes, chiggers, etc. They also get spider bites. This section does not address venomous bites, as that is an entirely different subject. Children tend to overreact to insect bites. Their skin swells and the bite often becomes hard and red, but not infected. My parents always told me it was because children are sweeter than adults. That is true in so many ways. I learned in residency that vitamin B1, in combination with the other B vitamins, gets into the skin and makes the child less appealing to insects.

However, I have also learned (from Prevention Magazine) that with any insect bite, a slice of onion works wonderfully. It does not matter what type of onion. Slice it and rub the slice on the bite until the juice is gone. It takes about one to three minutes. It is best done when the bite is fresh, but it can be done even a day or so later. The enzyme in the onion either draws out the toxin or neutralizes it, and the bite does not swell or itch. I found it originally for bee stings. The onion will also draw out the stinger from a bee sting, if it remains in the skin.

I have used this in bee stings, wasp stings, mosquito bites, spider bites, and ant bites. The results are consistent and amazing. I even had a patient call from Puerto Rico many years ago to tell me her child had a spider bite that had swollen and covered most of the child's thigh. I told her to use the onion, and by morning, the swelling was reduced to the size of a quarter. I used it on my finger when I had a wasp sting. It took ten minutes and three onion slices, but still the pain was gone and the swelling was one-fourth the size it would have been without this intervention.

This is not to be used for animal or human bites.

Migraines

Migraine headaches are vascular headaches that are intense and debilitating. They can occur at any age and are more common when there is a family history. They can be preceded by an aura of taste, a visual flash of lights, or even an auditory sensation. Basilar migraines can be signaled by weakness of one side of the body or slurred speech. The cause is still unknown.

There are several types of migraines. A **classic** migraine has an aura and a **common** migraine does not. **Basilar** migraines commonly have neurological symptoms associated with them like weakness on one side

A migraine generally has several characteristics. It is bad enough to interrupt daily activity. It can cause nausea and vomiting, sonophobia (sound bothers the patient) or photophobia (light bothers). Less than 50 percent of patients will have an aura preceding the headache. Migraines can also signal an underlying seizure disorder.

Migraines are common in children, but are most common in women ages thirty-five to forty-five years old. They affect more than eleven million Americans. Thirty-one percent of patients experience more than six migraines a year and do not seek medical help. Compliance with prophylaxis is not high (my experience is that most people do not want to take everyday medicine for "headaches"). Many patients do not find the preventive medicine effective enough to continue.

Many patients with migraines have low magnesium in their serum, saliva, red blood cells, monocytes, and CSF (cerebrospinal fluid). Calcium levels are normal. Hence, magnesium supplementation and riboflavin (B2) can help alleviate migraine frequency and intensity.

In the emergency department, magnesium, 1 gram, given IV over fifteen minutes can help terminate migraines in the acute situation.

1. New onset headaches (HA) and HA that wake a person at night are red flags that require further workup.

2. Headaches with a vertiginous (make one dizzy) component, require an EEG (brain wave test or electroencephalogram).

   There can be headache, visual scotomata (spots in front of the eyes or defects in peripheral vision), nausea, and vomiting. A headache with these characteristics can be a presentation of benign epilepsy.

3. Cluster headaches have horrible lancinating (stabbing) pain.

4. Basilar migraines often present with hemiparesis (weakness on one side of the body) or syncope (fainting). They *always* need prophylaxis.

5. The "common migraine" is the most common, and often in children does not have an aura. It is most often in the front of the head and on both sides. Patients with common migraine can have sonophobia (sound bothers them), nausea, and vomiting. There is usually a positive family history although not as often as we would expect.

6. Migraines are thought to have an inflammatory basis, and there is a release of inflammatory neuropeptides from the Trigeminal (fifth cranial nerve) ganglia.

7. Causes can be diverse and some are serious. Tumors, AVMs (Arterio-venous malformation), epilepsy, pregnancy, iron deficiency anemia, thyroid, parathyroid, obesity, and Arnold Chiari malformation can all cause severe headaches. The good news is that there is generally not a serious underlying cause.

8. There is an underlying hormonal cause in most women. Check out the website www.migrainecures. com.

Common Migraine

1. A detailed family history is necessary.
2. A physical exam with attention to nervous system exam is required.

3. "What makes it better? What makes it worse?" Be aware of modalities. Does the patient prefer a hot pack or a cold pack? Must the patient lie down or sleep it off? What does she think triggered it? What is her diet like? Stress level? Sleep patterns? How often does the patient have ANY headache?

4. ALL headaches are considered migraines once a patient is identified as a *migraineur*. So a "migraine" becomes a HA that has a pain level of nine to ten but lesser headaches are still part of the problem. The goal is to be headache free.

5. Medical treatment hopes to achieve a goal of decreased frequency and intensity; a reduction of 75 percent is considered successful. If a patient has a headache more than once a week, he or she needs prophylaxis (daily medicine to prevent them).

6. Everyone gets an imaging study (CT or MRI scan of the head) at some point. I prefer to do it early in the evaluation.

7. Traditional medical therapy is considered abortive (simply get rid of it); rescue (you are having trouble with abortive); and prophylactic (you have too many headaches).

8. Abortive Therapy
    a. Reglan has anti-migraine and anti-nausea properties. Use 5 mg for the small ones and 10 mg for the big ones (children, not HA). This is only prescribed by a physician.
    b. Triptans
        2. Accert, Zomig, Imitrex = quick acting
        3. Relpax is medium acting
        4. Frova and Amerge are longer acting
        5. Accert has the least cardiac affects.
        6. Zomig comes as a chewable.
            All the short acting ones give the "rush" of vasodilation. It is a gross feeling. Triptans are

used in patients eleven years old and up, and are prescribed by your physician.

c. Midrin and Fioricet are next if the Triptans are not working.

d. Motrin or Alleve (200-400 mg) can boost the effect of the Triptans.

e. DHE=Migranol which is a nasal spray. DHE=dihydroergotamine and is given via an IV in the hospital. It is 90 percent effective. Inpatient therapy will also use Depakote, Haldol, and Mellaril concurrently to break the severe and recalcitrant headache.

f. Steroids for four to five days can also help.

g. Ambien, so the patient can SLEEP.

All of the above are to be prescribed only by your healthcare provider or neurologist.

9. PROPHYLAXIS

a. Elavil at bedtime. This can be titrated up over two weeks. It is 75 to 80 percent effective. This is also a good choice if the patient is not sleeping well.

b. Calcium Channel Blockers and Propranolol have fallen into disfavor because of too many side effects.

c. SSRIs (Selective Serotonin Reuptake Inhibitors) are 50 percent effective and are the first choice if there is anxiety or stress-related symptoms. Fifty milligrams of Zoloft at bedtime is a first choice.

d. Antiepileptic (prescribed by a neurologist)

1. Topamax once daily for migraines, and twice daily for seizures. Twenty-five to fifty milligrams at bedtime. If 200 mg offers no relief, then higher doses will not work.. Topamax is an appetite suppressant. Side effects include word finding difficulties. No blood work is needed.

2. Neurontin, once daily for migraines, and twice daily for seizures. Starting dose is 100-300 mg and can be titrated up. Once the patient is on 900 mg with no effect, quit trying. It also comes as a liquid. It can cause irritability, tremor, dry mouth, and meanness.

3. Depakote has its place in therapy. I have seen it work miracles in some patients. Side effects can include hair loss, weight gain, and acne. Liver functions have to be monitored.

4. Zonogram has a side effect that can include enuresis.

5. Periactin is for little ones, and helps prevent allergies. Can be given twice daily. It is also an appetite stimulant. It does not work in those who are over eight to nine years old. Use one-half tab (4 mg tab) or one-half teaspoon (2 mg/5 ml).

All of the above are to be prescribed by your healthcare provider or neurologist. Every medicine has its benefits and its drawbacks. Your physician will discuss what is the best option for your child.

10. Triggers—find them and avoid them. The best medicine is to avoid the triggers—nuts, red wine, aged cheeses (cheddar comes to mind), chocolate, perfumes or strong smells, stress, fatigue, MSG, dairy, lima beans, fava beans, fresh breads and donuts (yeast products), processed meats, hot dogs, and meats with nitrates). Spicy foods are a huge trigger. Change in weather can also precipitate migraines, as can stress and insomnia. The best way to find your trigger is to keep a journal. When headaches strike, reviewing the journal can help you discover if there are patterns of foods or events that occur prior to the onset of the headache.

Chinese medicine has a very helpful way of looking at migraines. Too much heat causes those triggered by spicy foods. Spicy foods hit the digestive tract and emit heat from the spices. Hot air rises to the head and a migraine develops. It is too much yang (which is masculine and hot in Chinese medicine. Yin is female and cool.) Avoiding spicy foods is the first step to reducing such migraines. Cooling foods like cucumber and pears can help diminish the heat and abort the headache. I have tried green apples in the past with good results. Lemon is also a cooling food, so lots of water with lemon also helps flush the system and cool the fire.

There are other kinds of migraine qualities in Chinese medicine. It is best to see an experienced Chinese medicine practitioner for further evaluation.

Chiropractic care can also help find triggers, keep the spinal column aligned, and minimize a migraine. I have known patients whose migraines disappeared with chiropractic care. I have had a migraine go from an eight to a two after an adjustment.

Muscles along the cervical spine can become intensely tight and trigger what is now called a cervical migraine. I personally do not care what you call it, because once it is on, it is a miserable experience, and all the treatments come into play. Just get it gone, so I can think, see, and live normally again.

Medication ABORTIVE Summary
1. Motrin
2. Reglan
3. Triptan, or Triptan + Motrin
4. Midrin
5. Fioricet
6. Neurologist

Prophylactic Medication
1. Elavil
2. SSRIs
3. Topamax

4. Neurontin
5. Zonogram
6. Periactin
7. Periactin
8. Vitamin B2 400 mcg a day (found as Riboflavin 5 phosphate)
9. Magnesium 250-400 mg a day
10. Calcium 400 mg a day
11. CoQ10-100mg/day
12. Numbers 8-11 are over the counter doses for patients over 10 years old. Vitamin D may also have anti-migraine and anti-inflammatory benefits. Check out www.migrainecures.com.

There are other treatments that do help with migraines in some patients. As stated above, chiropractic care can have an amazing affect, as can Craniosacral therapy. Acupuncture, Chinese herbal therapies, homeopathy, yoga, and Pilates can also help reduce migraines.

The most important lesson I have learned <u>is to take medication early</u> (if I have been foolish enough to eat something that triggered one). Migraines are more easily aborted when you are aggressive in abortive therapy. Once the headache gets away from you, it is a one to three day ordeal depending on your severity scale. There is little need to suffer and much need to determine triggers, avoid them, and find which preventive therapies work.

Molluscum Contagiosum

Molluscum contagiosum is a warty-looking growth that occurs commonly on children. It is caused by a wart-like virus (yet unnamed and undiscovered but undoubtedly in the wart family). It tends to congregate on the sides of the body in the axillary area. It can spread to the arms, legs, buttocks, genitalia, neck, and rarely the face. The bigger ones look like they have a center, and indeed they do. Squeezing this center out causes the lesion to become red and inflamed, but not infected, and then it heals. Like warts, once one gets irritated and leaves, often the smaller friends leave with it.

It is a benign condition. It will disappear on its own, eventually. We do not refer patients to a dermatologist for this condition, as the treatment is more painful than the problem.

Molluscum is easily treated with homeopathic pellets—Thuja 30c or 200c daily for thirty days.

Tea tree oil applied directly with a Q-tip may also help. Tea tree oil can sting on young skin, so keeping it only on the molluscum is helpful.

Duct tape can also work. Put a small piece of duct tape on the biggest one at night. In the morning, rip it off. It is the non-gentle act of ripping it off that irritates the bump, and that makes it inflamed so it will storm off. This works in older children, but probably not so much in the little ones. I tell parents you'll be able to do it once, and then your child will avoid you whenever they see a roll of tape in your hand.

I have had excellent outcomes using the Thuja and duct tape as first line treatments, and not necessarily together!

Mononucleosis

Mono is one of my personal favorites as an illness. It is caused by Epstein Barr Virus, which is a member of the Herpes clan. It is common, common, common. About 75 percent of children will have this before age five. In children that young, it looks like a cold.

It has affectionately been called the "kissing disease" because a lot of teenagers get it that way. It is transmitted via saliva. I had a whole football team get it once from sharing a water bottle. This is one time that being a tiny bit germophobic is good! The worst case I have seen was a teenage girl who was very hygienically aware and got it from sharing ketchup with her best friend. They did not share fries, just the ketchup they dipped them in.

It often presents with a nasty sore throat and tests positive for strep. If in twenty four to forty eight hours the patient is not   feeling better, testing for mono should be done as it is often positive. Mono is interesting in that the patient must be sick five days before you can test. There is a short window during the illness, between days five and ten, when you can get a positive IgM level which means that the mono is acutely, right now positive. After that window, only IgG antibodies become positive, indicating the mono may be convalescing or has occurred sometime in the past. Mono can also present with fevers up to 104 degrees. Fever can persist for three to four weeks in rare cases.

Mono definitely affects the immune system. The teenage or adult patient may be extraordinarily fatigued and unable to make it past a half day at school. They may need to sleep eighteen hours a day. The liver and spleen may be swollen. The viral infection in the liver leads to swelling or liver inflammation (also known as hepatitis). The hepatitis goes away as the mono heals. However, there can be NO contact sports for three weeks while the liver and spleen are healing. A sudden hit to the abdomen can cause the spleen to rupture, and that requires a stay in the hospital.

Medical treatment for mono is limited. It is a virus. Bed rest, plenty of fluids, eating, and reassurance are what we have to offer. Mono can resolve in a few weeks or can have a prolonged course that takes months for the patient to recover.

Echinacea is a good blood cleanser and often makes a big difference. I use a "mono" tea from a Chinese herbalist that helps the body heal rapidly. My best case was a college student who came home with mono. The patient was so tired she was unable to stand up in the shower. Liver enzymes were elevated. I believed she would be home for a month. She took the mono tea, and in <u>one</u> week, her liver enzymes were 50 percent better and her energy was up 70 percent. She returned to school after ten days, and not the month I predicted!

When the tonsils and nodes are so swollen that there is potential obstruction of the airway or difficulty breathing, a short course of steroids can be prescribed. At this point, the steroids are necessary to decrease the inflammatory process so breathing is not hindered. It is not desirable to give steroids in most febrile illnesses as they do suppress the immune system, which in the case of mono, is already under fire. There has been some concern that is not yet proven that steroid use in mono may be linked to lymphoma later. We prescribe steroids only when absolutely necessary.

The mono tea helps heal the body and rids itself of the illness. Steroids just treat the symptoms. Mono is better treated with alternative medicine therapies, while strep throat is still better treated with antibiotics. Mono tea can be obtained through my office.

MRSA

MRSA is Methicillin Resistant Staphylococcal Aureus. It is a skin bacterium that has developed resistance to the antibiotic Methicillin and the penicillin family in general.

The news has done an excellent job broadcasting information that increases fear by focusing only on how deadly MRSA can be. MRSA does cause serious infections and can lead to death if it invades the body and takes hold. Usually it causes skin infections and boils. It originally was found only in hospitals and now is in the community. "Community" acquired MRSA has become quite "smart" and actually can cause worse illness than MRSA found in the hospitals. It is important (like everything else) to be aware and to take preventive measures with this germ. I do not want to diminish how severe this disease can be, but rather put it in perspective. There are many "bad" germs out there, but we do not hear about all of them every day except when they hit the headlines.

Any "boil" or skin infection that comes on fast and hard needs to be seen by a physician. Any "boil" near the nose needs to be seen as well. I believe that if the infection is near a mucous membrane it may have the potential to invade the body more easily. The definitive treatment is incision and drainage (lancing it). The infection heals rapidly and often does not need antibiotics when treated this way. Your physician may give you Bactroban (mupiricin) to apply topically **and** in your nose. A new topical cream, Altabax, works even better on the topical lesions. MRSA is often carried in the nose of patients who have recurrent infections. It can become a "family affair," so once one family member develops a MRSA infection, anyone else who has an infected sore needs to be seen and the assumption is MRSA until proven otherwise. The good news is that it will not plague you forever.

Otitis Media (Ear Infections)

Otitis media is the fancy Latin name for middle ear infection. It is extremely common in children (much more so in the last twenty years than when we parents were growing up, but lots of things have changed in this time. Why not ear infections?).

The most common germ-causing ear infections used to be Haemophilus Influenza. That has decreased because of the HIB shot. (H. influenza also causes meningitis, and H. Flu meningitis has decreased to almost nothing since the inception of the HIB vaccine in 1985). Strep pneumonia became the more common cause of ear infections, causing one out of three of the infections. Viral infection is the cause of two-thirds of ear infections.

Prevnar is the newest vaccine that provides immunity to deter infections caused by strep pneumonia. It has helped decrease the number of ear infections caused by strep pneumonia, but it has more importantly helped reduce <u>invasive</u> infections like pneumonia and meningitis from this bacteria. Strep pneumonia can be a vicious germ. It causes whatever organ it settles in to become filled with pus. I read that this germ caused the death of Jim Henson, the Muppet Man. He had pneumonia. He had been ill for three days with flu-like symptoms; by the time he went to the hospital, the infection had most likely filled his lungs with pus and he had become septic, meaning the infection had entered his blood stream and was everywhere. He was only fifty-three when he died. This particular germ seems to be found frequently in day-care facilities as well. It can cause mild infection or serious infection. Our goal with the Prevnar vaccine is obviously to prevent serious infection. The latest information involving this vaccine illustrates one negative consequence of vaccines. The Prevnar covers seven strains or serotypes of streptococcus pneumonia. One of them is strain 19F. Its "cousin," 19A, is not in this vaccine and has found the opportunity to increase in prevalence and simultaneously develop antibiotic resistance.

Ear infections can come on very rapidly or can occur more slowly at the end of a cold that has been ongoing for several days. An ear infection often does NOT need antibiotic therapy.

Treatment suggestions include:

1. Acetaminophen or ibuprofen for discomfort
2. Garlic and willow drops (or garlic and mullein or garlic and goldenseal) two drops, two to four times a day. This alone can be all the child needs.
3. Homeopathic remedies also work wonders. M. Panos; *Homeopathy at Home* or Ullman and Cummings book, *Everybody's Guide to Homeopathic Medicine* can be great resources for simple infections that can be treated at home.

   The most common homeopathic remedy that I use for ear infections is **Pulsatilla** in a dose of 200c. Children with earaches may have been sick a day or two and now are very whiney, clingy, pitiful, and cry over the least little thing. Their thirst may be down from normal. Their symptoms may be worse around dinnertime, and they are fussier. This is a great children's remedy and works well. Dissolve two pellets in water and give one ounce two to three times a day for two to three days. When it is right, there is symptom relief within one to two hours.

   Belladonna 200c works if the child wakes suddenly in the night screaming and pulling or complaining about the right ear. Its key symptoms are sudden onset, red, hot, and throbbing pain. Dissolve two pellets in water and give one ounce two to three times a day for two to three days. When it is right, there is symptom relief within one to two hours.
4. There are other remedies covered in the books mentioned (*Homeopathy at Home* and *Everybody's Guide to Homeopathic Medicine*). Beyond this, the patient needs to be seen by their physician.

5. Antibiotics are often used when the pain is unbearable and the child has a fever with the infection. In twenty-one years of practice, I have found that with uncomplicated ear infection that three to four days of antibiotics is all that is needed to clear the infection. (This means there are no other significant illnesses like strep throat or pneumonia in conjunction with the ear infection.) This is different from the standard ten days that is recommended. I am simply telling you what has worked repeatedly with no relapse of ear infection for me for many years.

6. Sometimes children need longer rounds of medical treatment, and there are still those who benefit from tubes after repeated ear infections.

7. In my practice, we have found that many children with repeated ear infections or those who continue to have them after tubes are put in have an underlying food allergy. Dairy is the number one suspect, and often stopping dairy products makes a HUGE difference in these patients' health.

8. Probiotics (good bacteria for the colon) are also helpful when a child has repeated infections. Bifidus Bifidobacterium is the kind that children up to age seven need. After age seven, Lactobacillus and Bifidus are needed. These bacteria keep balance in the gut and there is some evidence that the synergistic relationship of balanced bacteria promotes good immune function. Perhaps these bacteria in proper balance make a natural antiviral called interferon. This antiviral would help our bodies kill invading viruses.

9. Fish oil (cod liver oil) is also very helpful in supporting the immune system. Cod liver oil is also rich in vitamin A and vitamin D.

Pharyngitis

Pharyngitis is an inflammation of the pharynx, or more simply put, sore throat. Sore throats are common, part of a simple cold, or can be more severe as in strep throat.

Viral sore throats typically are scratchy or can feel raw. Sometimes it hurts to swallow and sometimes it does not. There are usually other symptoms associated like runny nose, a slight cough, and feeling tired.

Strep throat is caused by Group A beta hemolytic strep. Usually it has a sudden onset. You wake up and feel a little scratchy throat and a few hours later you feel like you got hit by a truck and swallowing becomes very painful. Strep is uncommon in children under two unless they are exposed to it via another family member or someone in day care.

There are seven typical symptoms that do not all have to be present:

1. Headache
2. Sore throat
3. Stomach ache
4. Rash
5. Fever
6. Vomiting
7. Diarrhea

Often when there are two or three of these symptoms, we will test for strep. The typical strep throat rash is a scarlet fever (scarlatinform) rash that starts in the groin. It is a solid red, sandpapery rash. It can spread all over the body. It is not typically itchy but can be. It looks like a mild sunburn, and like sunburn, may peel during the healing stages.

The rash is caused by a virus that gets into the bacteria and causes it to produce a toxin that then causes the rash.

Treatment of strep throat is still penicillin (or a cephalosporin for penicillin-allergic patients). It can be treated homeopathically, but that is only in conjunction with antibiotics. Some strains of strep are "rheumatogenic" and can cause rheumatic fever if the strep goes untreated. There is NO sense in taking that chance. Strep is still very sensitive to penicillins and therefore is treated uniformly with antibiotics. Strep requires 10 full days of treatment.

A rapid strep test in the office is very accurate when strep bacteria are present. It is more reliable when the patient has been sick a day or two. Sometimes when the patient has been sick only one day, and the symptoms are mild; there is not enough bacteria replication to get a positive test. Sometimes strep presents so classically it is easy to diagnose. On physical exam, in a classic case, the throat is beefy red and there are red dots (petechiae) on the roof of the mouth. The tonsils may be swollen and there may be pus (exudate) on them. The cervical (neck) lymph nodes may be swollen and tender as well. There may or may not be a rash as described above. Strep is so sensitive to penicillin that after twenty-four hours on antibiotics the patient feels 100 percent better and is no longer contagious. Patients may return to school or work at this point (I know this is a disappointment to many of you).

Viral pharyngitis may also have swollen tonsils, exudate, and tender nodes, but the strep test will be negative. Gargling with salt water (a gold standard, tried and true, and it makes me throw up) or a solution of half-peroxide, half-Listerine (or whatever mouthwash you prefer) helps soothe the pain of swallowing. The peroxide (H2O2) does the work and the mouthwash makes it tolerable. If you gargle with peroxide alone (I tried it), it feels like all the liquid has been sucked out of your mouth and you gag. It's gross. I recommend Listerine because the TV commercials do say "Nine out of ten doctors recommend Listerine for their patients." I wasn't sure I wanted to be number ten on that list.

In summary, sore throats are either viral or bacterial. The most common sore throat bacteria are group A strep and requires antibiotic therapy. If strep is not present, symptomatic treatment will help ease the discomfort.

Probiotics

I have mentioned this word several times. Probiotics ("for living organisms") are beneficial BACTERIA for our intestines. At birth, we are supposed to be colonized with Bifidus bifidobacterium, and then as we mature, other bacteria colonize our intestinal environment and work synergistically to create a harmonious synchrony of function. (Oh, doesn't that sound great?) What it means is that we are supposed to have bacteria in our gut and the bacteria work together to digest food, enhance our immune system, and to create and remove toxins our body does not need. Typically, we have Bifidus, Lactobacillus species, E.coli, and a mix of other bacteria that create a friendly environment.

When this balance is upset through poor nutrition or disease, there is an imbalance. Then unfriendly or pathogenic bacteria seize the opportunity to take over (a hostile takeover as it were) and wreak further havoc. This imbalance can manifest as diarrhea, constipation, rashes, general immune weakness, or a host of other problems. Replenishing beneficial bacteria and restoring balance can alleviate a lot of symptoms.

Studies are clearly showing that probiotics help in acute infectious diarrhea. They lessen the course of illness. I have seen probiotics in the newborn alleviate colic and treat what appears to be early eczema. When used with antibiotics, they can prevent antibiotic associated diarrhea. They help with candidiasis (yeast overgrowth) and small bowel overgrowth. Two strains of beneficial bacteria that have been well studied are Culturelle and *Lactobacillus reuteri*. I use these in children over three on a regular basis. Children under three do well with a single source of *Bifidus bifidobacterium.*

There is another probiotics out now called Florastor. This is a good YEAST—Saccharomyces boulardii. It is not a bacteria; it is a probiotic. It is "good" yeast that secretes a sugary coat of mannose in the intestine and then attracts "bad" bacteria, binds them, and allows for them to be pooped out. It is excellent in travelers' diarrhea, antibiotic associated diarrhea and in chronic bowel conditions like Crohn's and ulcerative colitis. Its presence allows the normal good bacteria to increase and restore balance. It is taken twice a day for ten days in acute infections and can be taken indefinitely in chronic illnesses. It is the SAME dose from two months to 200 years old (in infants and adults) —250 mg twice a day.

I am certain there will be more information and usage of probiotics in the future. It is becoming more and more imperative to avoid the use of antibiotics in mild illness and to help the body's own immune system heal minor infections. A healthy immune system also will prevent serious illness

Scars

Everyone gets a cut or laceration that needs stitches at some point, and everyone has a scar of some sort. Some scars we are proud of and some not so much. Different parts of the body heal better than others, and some people heal better than others do.

The face and the pelvic area are rich in blood supply and tend to heal faster and better than other parts of the body. The legs heal the slowest because they are dependent or hanging down all day and the blood supply is not as rich. It is harder for blood to flow against gravity or uphill, and hence it can take longer for leg wounds to heal, and they may not heal as nicely as those on the face or in the pelvic area.

The face is very forgiving because of its abundant blood supply. I have seen cuts that needed stitches and did not get them as well as some poorly repaired face wounds. After six months, both healed in thin lines that were barely noticeable. So when in doubt, wait. Give it six months. Besides, even wounds that we know will need revision by a plastic surgeon must wait six months before the surgeon will consider repair.

Wounds that need suturing require different lengths of time that the sutures need to be left in for proper healing to occur.

Face sutures come out after four to five days. This avoids the old "railroad track" scars from yesteryear, again, because the face heals so quickly. Wounds on the arms, legs, and back have stitches left in nine to ten days for maximum healing, and to prevent spreading of the suture line.

After the stitches come out, lacerations often have hardness under them called *fibrosis*. This scar tissue reorganizes over time and smoothes out so the scar is barely visible. We recommend using cocoa butter, shea butter, or Schmoove (obtained through our office). Rubbing the wound every day with gentle massage helps break up the fibrosis and speeds the recovery process as well as reduces the appearance of the scar.

Some wounds will develop extra scar tissue, which is also called hypertrophy or keloid. This is common in African Americans and in families with this tendency. Areas that are *high use* areas like the back, legs, and parts of the arm are more prone to keloid. It is difficult to avoid keloid formation at times.

The treatment of keloid is basically to prevent it.

One can also use Thiocinnamum (homeopathic tincture) to soften the keloid. Schmoove and Revive (again from Si Jin Bao) are Chinese herbal creams that make a marked difference in reducing keloid formation. It is best to prevent keloid, if we can, rather than try to deal with it after it has formed. Over the counter Mederma also can help reduce scar formation and may help prevent keloid if used early.

If a keloid has been formed, despite all the best efforts to prevent its formation, the scar can be injected with steroids to decrease the size and flatten it out.

Sunburn

This should be a one sentence article—Do not ever get sunburned!

Many people do get sunburned every year. It is more likely for a person to get burned in tropical climates. In summer in Florida, it is so HOT and humid that you can get burned in thirty minutes during peak hours of sun, especially if you are without sunscreen. <u>There is no glory in getting a tan. Tanning IS sun damage.</u> Sun damage <u>accumulates</u> over the years and leads to skin cancer.

Some sun is good. We receive Vitamin D from the sun, but burning is <u>never</u> healthy, and burning in your adolescent years sets the stage for skin cancer as early as your twenties.

First and foremost, prevent sunburns.

1. Children under six months old cannot wear sunscreen. Keep them out of the sun during peak hours. Be sure they are not out in the heat for long hours as children can "bake." Heat and light are reflected off concrete, sand, and water.

2. Wear sunblock <u>and</u> sunscreen. There are many good brands of sunblock and sunscreen available. Blue Lizard and Arbonne are two brands I like.

3. Wear protective clothing. There are many companies making sun protective clothing and hats. The tight weave helps prevent the penetration of UV rays through the clothing.

4. Remember, if you are in the water, reapply sunscreen and sunblock every one to two hours, as it washes off.

5. Remember that cloudy days are more than capable of causing significant sunburns. Cloudy days result in worse sunburns because people are deceived into thinking they are not getting sun and stay out longer than they would on a bright sunny day.

6. If you or your child has a very short haircut or is bald, wear sunscreen or a hat, as your scalp <u>will</u> burn. (Been there, done that and it was MISERABLE!)

If you have a serious lapse in judgment and do get burned:

1. Ibuprofen works wonders. So does Vitamin C 250-500 mg twice a day.
2. Aloe gel or aloe plant is cool and soothing.
3. Lavender oil spray can reduce the pain.
   Homeopathic remedies Apis, Cantharis, and Urtica urens (30c or 200c) can also decrease the pain of minor sunburn. Dissolve two pellets in water and give one ounce two to three times a day for two to three days. When it is right, there is symptom relief within one to two hours.
4. Schmoove can also work wonders as it decreases redness, pain, and blistering.

If you go beyond judgment, lapse into foolishness, and get a second degree burn:

1. You will be in severe pain. You will blister! You will peel in sheets. You will have trouble sleeping for several nights. You may have to visit the emergency department nearest you.
2. Medically, such sunburns are treated with ibuprofen and prednisone to decrease the inflammation, and Silvadene (cream for burns). Aloe can also work.
   The homeopathic remedy <u>Cantharis</u>, if given early, can actually help prevent blistering. <u>Apis</u> is excellent for the intense pain and stinging. It feels better with cooling and worse with touch. Dissolve two pellets in water and give one ounce two to three times a day for two to three days. When it is right, there is symptom relief within one to two hours.

3. We recently had an experience with a ten-year-old playing on a boogie board for three hours, without sunscreen, in the sun, at the beach at the surf line. The child developed second-degree sunburn with big yellow blisters on the back and chest and was unable to wear a shirt because of the pain of anything touching the skin. This child could not sleep for two nights because of the severe pain. We used Cantharis, Aloe, and spray Schmoove. The combination brought the redness and pain down within <u>hours</u>. This child had to drink a lot of fluids because with sunburn (ANY burns) there is increased water loss from the body, and it is important to stay hydrated to prevent infection.

4. We could not use Silvadene because the patient would have to be wrapped in gauze and could tolerate nothing touching the skin. With the combination of remedies, herbal tea, and the spray Schmoove, this patient was 100 percent better in less than twenty-four hours. (After three days of misery where aloe, Motrin, and other over-the-counter measures did not work).The skin will still peel, but this patient healed without scarring or infection. Schmoove was the miracle cream.

We do not advise anyone to get this sunburned, ever! Prevention is everything. THINK! Do not let your children leave the house without applying sunscreen first for a day outside! Sunscreen needs about thirty minutes to soak in before it can be protective. Wear a hat and appropriate clothing in a boat, at the beach, or skiing, etc!

EVERYONE feels horrible when this kind of thing happens, and it is 100 percent preventable!

Warts

Warts are a skin problem caused by a virus and are most commonly found in young people but can occur at any age. Common areas of occurrence are the face, hands, elbows, and knees. They can be flat or "verrucous," meaning bumpy like a cauliflower.

Plantar warts occur on the bottoms of the feet. They are actually regular warts, but because one stands on his feet all day, the constant pressure makes the wart grow inward rather than outward. Plantar warts can become painful as they can feel like little rocks in the foot. Putting pressure on them hurts, and if they are big enough, walking can be painful.

Venereal warts are found on the genitals or around the anus in both sexes. Warts usually disappear spontaneously. Fortunately there is a wide range of treatments, including local application of chemicals, removal with a curette, and electrocautery (burning).

The medical name for warts is verruca.

Typical treatments are traditionally freezing or burning off the wart. I do not recommend burning, as in my experience, the warts recur and double in number. Freezing with liquid nitrogen is the most commonly accepted medical treatment. Sometimes it can take several treatments to completely get rid of a wart.

There are alternative therapies for treating warts.

All remedies are dosed as follows: Dissolve two pellets in water and give one ounce two to three times a day for twenty to thirty days.

1. Causticum 200c potency works well. Take two pellets one to two times a day for up to thirty days. This is for warts on the hands, especially around the fingernails.

2. Thuja 200c also works well for warts. It is ideal for plantar warts, and again is administered two pellets daily for thirty days. Sometimes it can take two to four months for the warts to completely disappear. However, that is better than the one to two years it can take if you do nothing.

3. Duct Tape is also a popular therapy. The army did a study and showed that duct tape is as effective as other treatment modalities. It smothers the wart. Cut a piece of duct tape to cover the wart and

then leave it on for three weeks. Some children are so busy that a single piece will not stay on for three weeks. No problem. Just keep replacing it as it peels off. The goal is to keep the wart covered and smothered. Often I will suggest picking the biggest wart because when the biggest one leaves, it will often take all its skeevy little wart friends with it.

4. Mangosteen is an antioxidant drink that is good for the immune system. I have had parents tell me that applying this topically for two weeks got rid of their child's wart.

5. Tea Tree Oil is another popular therapy. Tea Tree Oil is a natural antifungal, anti bacterial, antiviral. Applied with a Q-tip topically as often as needed, it can also speed the healing of a wart.

6. C-Herb is a combination topical herb that can cause a wart to go away. This can be found on the Internet or in select health food stores.

7. I have not yet tried Schmoove on warts, but Schmoove is "nutrition for the skin" and can help any skin condition. It is a topical Chinese herbal cream and should be able to make a wart disappear after a few weeks of use.

8. Black Ointment and Pau D'Arco following Tea Tree Oil can also eliminate warts. The tea tree oil kills the virus and the other two speed the skin's repair.

9. Oregano Oil is a naturally potent antibacterial and antifungal oil. Rub a drop on the wart twice daily, and it should disappear within a few weeks. (Don't hold me to the timetable. It is an estimate.)

10. Cider Vinegar can also remove warts. Applying a cotton ball soaked in cider vinegar and taping it to the wart overnight is supposed to kill the virus. Do this nightly until the wart is gone.

11. I am sure there are other methods that are safe and effective to get rid of ugly warts. These are a few and are painless alternatives to traditional freezing of warts. All methods are viable and good ways to get rid of unpleasant and/or unsightly warts.

12. If warts recur despite therapy, then it is probably a good idea to boost the immune system so it is not so susceptible to warts or viral infections in general.

Chapter Four

Homeopathy and Health Pearls

There are many good practitioners who practice alternative medicine. It is more accepted in the Northeast and on the West Coast of the United States, so it is easier to locate practitioners in those areas.

There are only 1,000 (approximately) homeopathic practitioners trained in the U.S., and very few of those are medical doctors. My training and bias are towards classical homeopathy as pioneered by Samuel Hahnemann, MD in the 1800s. Classical homeopathy is based on three principles:

1. Law of Similars. This is the cornerstone of homeopathy. *Similia similibus curentur* means let likes be cured by likes. Any substance that causes symptoms in a healthy individual can heal a person experiencing similar symptoms.
2. Law of the single dose. In classical homeopathy, a detailed history is taken and a single medicine is sought to cover the totality of all symptoms.
3. Law of minimum dose. Because the body's own healing powers are so strong, often a single dose of a single remedy is needed to stimulate the healing process.

Constantine Hering was another brilliant homeopath and we still use *Hering's Law of Cure.* "Homeopaths define health as a state of freedom existing on three interrelated levels—the physical, the emotional, and the mental. A healthy person experiences physical vitality and freedom from physiological malfunction, emotional peace, freedom of expression, and mental clarity with creativity. The most serious symptoms affect the deeper, more vital parts of the person. When evaluating a patient's overall state of health, the homeopath views the mental state as most important, followed by the emotional state, and then the physical state" (*Everybody's Guide to Homeopathic Medicine,* Ullman and Cummings: *1997, p.12).*

The body also heals from the inside out and from top to bottom. It arranges its organs in a hierarchy from most important to least important. That hierarchy is as follows: Brain, Heart, Endocrine, Liver, Lung, Kidney, Bone, Muscle, and Skin. In the healing process, deeper issues will improve first and some of the more superficial problems may temporarily worsen.

In acute illnesses, remedies are often prescribed three times a day for two to three days only. When one has selected the correct remedy in an acute illness, the patient can expect to be at least 30 percent better in the first eight hours. If not, it is not the correct remedy and more information is needed.

People only become ill when their immune defenses are weakened, making them susceptible to illness. Grief, stress, malnutrition, drugs, and lack of sleep are examples of things that can make us susceptible and allow germs to gain a foothold and cause illness.

Homeopathic remedies are made from over 2,000 natural plants, animal, and mineral products. The remedies are prepared in specialized pharmacies by a process of dilution and succussion that increases potency. Many remedies are made from recognizable toxic elements, like arsenic and mercury. Through the process of dilution, there is no molecular substance left in the homeopathic remedy, rendering it non-toxic to the physical body. At this point, it becomes an instrument to stimulate the body to heal itself.

Allopathic medicines combat disease by actually suppressing symptoms. Antibiotics are necessary in many infections to kill harmful bacteria. After the infection is controlled, the body finishes the job. Other medicines, like steroids, can create other problems by suppressing symptoms, driving the illness deeper into the body. A great example of this concept is eczema and asthma. Traditional medical models recognize both disorders as part of an allergy march. We know that infants with eczema often develop asthma later. Chronic use of steroid creams can suppress eczema symptoms, driving the problem from the skin, deeper into the lungs and hence developing asthma. If we can treat the eczema and find the root cause with alternative therapies, it is reasonable to think we could actually prevent some children from developing asthma.

Combination remedies have become very popular, and classically trained homeopaths do not like them. The concept is to combine low potency remedies together by including several of the most common ones that are indicated in an acute illness. Then the hope is that one of them will be right and stimulate healing. There are a few combination remedies that are effective and useful in certain conditions, but overall, the principle is flawed. Classically trained homeopaths view the combination remedy in a similar fashion as a medical doctor would view combining five or six common antibiotics together and giving that combination to a patient in hopes that one of them covered the problem.

Most classically trained homeopaths in the U.S. have DNBHE, D Hom, and HomD after their names.

When seeking a Chinese herbalist or acupuncturist, it is important to find one who has completed a traditional three-year course in acupuncture and Chinese medicine. Many MDs can take a 200-hour course in acupuncture and then practice acupuncture. This is an abbreviated course that is geared ultimately towards alleviating symptoms rather than effecting cures by tracking the source of disease.

ALL disease is caused by a breach in the energetic body. We are all pummeled every day by germs, dirt, emotional issues, trauma, and structural misalignments, yet not everyone gets sick. A person becomes ill only when he is susceptible. Germs do not cause disease; they are merely opportunistic when there is a breach in the immune system from things like malnutrition, grief, or a simple overwhelming load of infection. Then the germ can gain a foothold and lead to sickness. It is not the germ alone that causes illness. It is the by-products or waste that it leaves in its wake. The body reacts to the waste products and that reaction leads to symptoms.

Ask around when you are seeking alternative therapy. Interview the practice and understand their philosophy. Most have the same underlying desire to root out the cause of the illness. It can take years to heal since it took years to get sick. Persistence and compliance will help in the healing process. In addition, the process can be different for every individual depending on the patient's individual problems. Most alternative practitioners do not file insurance. It can be a little expensive but in the long run saves thousands of dollars in treating chronic debilitating degenerative illnesses.

Basic Homeopathy

Read the text *Homeopathic Medicine at Home* by M. Panos or *Everybody's Guide to Homeopathic Medicine* by Dana Ullman and Stephen Cummings.

Calcarea Carbonica is a great remedy for children. It is commonly used for fears (in general), and definitely used for night terrors and nightmares. Dosing is 200c two times a day for seven to ten days. It can be used for recurrent ear infections and constipation (especially if the child is happy when constipated).

Arsenicum Album is a remedy used very commonly. It is number one for food poisoning or for symptoms that are like food poisoning that cause <u>vomiting and diarrhea</u>. You do not have to have food poisoning to have those symptoms. It is also good for asthma, and coughs that are better sitting up and that tend to be aggravated between midnight to 2:00 a.m. Symptoms may also include burning pains (anywhere) that are made better with heat applications. (Burning pain; better heat.) The patient wants to sip drinks (as opposed to gulping them) and can be anxious and restless (the restlessness is because the person cannot get away from his pain or discomfort and keeps moving from place to place even though he is exhausted). Dosing is 200c, three times a day for three to four days.

Bryonia is great for the flu. Patients needing this remedy have a GRUMPY attitude, like a bear. They like to be left alone. They like to splint their sore parts. If there is a headache, the patient will hold his head so it does not move. Symptoms are worse with the slightest movement and tend to get worse as the day goes on. Symptoms can peak around 9:00 p.m. Dosing is 200c three times a day for three to four days. This remedy is also great for sprains and strains, and GREAT for whiplash injuries, especially when used early.

Gelsemium is also used for the flu. Specific symptoms to look for that indicate the remedy will work are "dull, dopey, droopy, and dizzy." Dosing is 200c three times a day for three to four days.

Oscillococcinum is found in all health food stores. It also helps with the flu. It is best used at the beginning of symptoms. Take every eight hours. It helps prevent the flu as well as treats its symptoms. Started early it can shorten the course of illness. Directions say use one vial three times a day. I have found that one capful of the "tinies" three times a day works as well as the entire vial. One pellet or one vial is a dose. Homeopathic remedies are not dosed the same as traditional medications.

Arnica is number one for trauma for any "hemorrhagic extravasations," i.e. bruising. Can be used after tooth extractions, tooth cleaning, birth, or any injury/illness involving bruising. Great for jet lag or if one is feeling "beat up." It can be used for old injuries as well. For example, when someone says they have NBWS (never been well since), or a specific injury, Arnica in high potency 1M or 10M (obtained from your practitioner) can still work for the past injury as well as alleviate the ongoing symptoms that have arisen as a result of that injury. Dosing is 30c or 200c three to four times a day for three to four days for acute injuries.

Pulsatilla is a favorite for kids! Symptoms include weepy, whiney, clingy, pitiful, better being held, better outside, worse at twilight (dinner time). Discharges are bland, goopy, and yellow. Thirst is decreased from the child's normal state. It is also good for problems that started at puberty (Never Been Well Since=NBWS puberty). For acute illness, it is 30c or 200c three to four times a day for three to four days. "NBWS" puberty needs a practitioner's involvement.

Rhus Toxicodendron is great for chicken pox. It stops the itching and speeds crusting over of the lesions. It is also used in sprains and strains, especially if one feels stiff initially, better first motion, and better warmth. This remedy is also useful with herpetic cold sores. Take 200c three times a day for three to four days.

Silica: Made from sand, it is an excellent remedy to prevent side effects from vaccinations. Typically, one dose of 200c after a shot will prevent side effects. It can be used two to three times a day for one to two days if desired. This remedy is very helpful when there is a history of bad reactions to vaccines (Thuja and Carcinosin also have that in common). Silica is also helpful in children who are not gaining weight despite a healthy appetite. Give Silica 1M weekly for four weeks. It seems to work very well 90 percent of the time. This potency is obtained from your practitioner.

Podophyllum is indicated in painless explosive diarrhea and/or vomiting. A great remedy to use when someone has rotavirus. Give 30c or 200c with each stool. Diarrhea subsides with each dose when it is the correct remedy. This is an excellent remedy for diarrhea in general. If it does not work, it simply is the wrong remedy, and more information is needed to find the better suited remedy.

Phosphorous is a great remedy for fears. It is well suited to symptoms of vomiting when with the vomiting they are thirsty for cold drinks and vomit within five minutes of drinking (as soon as liquid warms in the stomach). Used a lot for cough and/or asthma and respiratory conditions where the child seems perfectly content but sounds awful and the parents are more worried than the child. Give 30c or 200c three times a day for two to three days. If the problem persists, see a practitioner. Phosphorous patients usually want <u>COLD</u> drinks and lots of them. This remedy is also good for clearing the after effects of anesthesia. Generally just one dose is needed after surgery to speed clearing of the fuzziness of anesthesia.

Apis is good for allergic reactions, including hives. There are often red, swollen, hot, stinging pains that are better cold and worse hot. A sore throat with those symptoms would respond to Apis. Dosing is 200c three times a day for one to two days.

Ignatia—1M is commonly used for acute grief reactions. The remedy helps the body heal and takes away the deep pain and hysteria. It provides a calming effect in the initial stages of grieving. Grief needs to be talked out. It should not be suppressed, as it will come out in some other way. I also recommend a picture album as a tool for healing. When a loved one dies, it is amazing to have your own album filled with pictures of that person. Then you can look through it whenever you miss the loved one. Initially you cry. Over time, though, the pictures remind you of all the happy times, and the grief subsides. This is especially helpful for children.

The following pearls are useful in our everyday practice. These are interesting facts I gathered from medical journal reading. Most of these pearls refer to adults, but I still found them informative, practical, and useful.

1. Tai Chi (supreme ultimate fist or boxing) is a martial arts form developed in the context of Chinese Taoism during the twelfth century. The traditional focus is on achieving mental balance, healthy longevity, and unity of mind and body. It is a low-impact exercise that is slow and coordinates deep breathing with graceful, meditative movements, meditation, and self-awareness. Tai Chi is definitely useful in preventing falls in the elderly.

2. PMS affects women in their thirties and forties. Three to eight percent of women are affected with PMDD (Premenstrual dysphoria disorder). Chaste Berry or Vitex in doses of 3.5 to 4.5 mg dried extract or 500 mg tablets (one or two) daily during the premenstrual cycle has been shown to decrease many symptoms of PMS, especially edema, moodiness and breast tenderness.

Vitex may also normalize bleeding patterns. Acupuncture can help alleviate many of these symptoms as well.

3. Journaling is the process of writing down emotional upheavals. It has been shown that physical and mental health improves when emotional events can be put into words via talking or writing. Putting feelings in to words removes them to the "outside" (externalizes) of our bodies and releases negativity. This release improves mental and immune health and can improve memory and cognitive function. The field of psycho-neuro-immunology explores how our mental and emotional health affects our immune system. The three are intrinsically connected.

   Patients with asthma and rheumatoid arthritis have noticed improved symptoms after writing about past stressful experiences.

   Patients with PTSD (post traumatic stress disorder) do slightly worse if they write about their experiences. They are not encouraged to journal.

   By writing about stressful events, they are "exposed", and repressed thoughts can move from subconscious to conscious where they can be organized and controlled. The therapy is the writing itself. It is private, No one has to read it if the patient so desires. When repressed thoughts are released, the mind processes from I and me to we and us, decreasing feelings of isolation and engendering connection with the community.

4. Echinacea does not relieve the symptoms of URI (upper respiratory infection) in children. Echinacea is in the daisy and ragweed family, so people with allergies to those plants may wish to avoid Echinacea. As an immune system modulator, it stimulates white cells to eat germs, as well as stimulating other monocytes and natural killer cells. It may increase interleukins, tumor necrosis factor, and interferon. Echinacea should not be used in autoimmune diseases like TB, SLE, MS, HIV (Tuberculosis, Systemic Lupus Erythematosis, Multiple Sclerosis, and Aids).

5. Andrographis (Indian Echinacea) is an excellent herb for treating the common cold (URI) in adults.
   Its mechanism of action is unknown.

It stimulates the immune system by increasing antibody activity and Macrophage phagocytosis (white cells eating germs).

i. It is an overall tonic

ii. It has been used as a cold remedy in Sweden for years.

The dose is 400 mg three times a day for URI symptoms.

It may exacerbate autoimmune disease.

6. Meditation is "intentional self-regulation of present awareness." Mindfulness meditation emphasizes detached observation of oneself engaged in a practice, such as breathing. Jon Kabat-Zinn (*Wherever You Go There You Are*) is the best author on this subject. Mindfulness meditation helps with chronic pain by breaking the connection between the sensory interpretation and the pain experience.. Studies show sustained physical and psychological benefits in chronic pain patients.

7. Cannabis (marijuana) use among youth has now been shown to have an increased risk of mental illness later in life, specifically psychosis and affective (mood) disorders.

8. Jet Lag is defined as fatigue, irritability, decreased concentration, decreased productivity, and sleep problems. The severity of symptoms depends upon how many time zones are crossed. (Eastward travel is more difficult than westward travel). It takes four to six days to establish normal sleep patterns after flying through six or more time zones.

Melatonin is synthesized in the pineal gland under the control of the circadian clock located in the hypothalamus. Body temp reaches its lowest between 4:00 and 5:00 a.m. when melatonin is highest.

Take 5 mg beginning at bedtime in the destination zone on the day of the flight and for two to seven days after. Do not take if you're on anticoagulants. Aspirin, Ibuprofen, and beta blockers can suppress your own endogenous melatonin release.

Usual dose for adults is 3 mg at bedtime for insomnia.

I have used this in children over the age of six in 1 mg doses at bedtime.

9. Antibacterial soaps do not reduce the risk for developing symptoms of infectious disease among generally healthy people. They do not affect viral illnesses at all. Plain soap and water work as well, if not better.

10. Acupuncture leads to persistent clinically important benefits in people with chronic headaches, especially migraines. In one study, acupuncture improved health-related quality of life at minimal additional cost.

11. COQ10 can be recommended to patients with Type 2 diabetes. It can be beneficial for vascular function and blood pressure. It can decrease effectiveness of warfarin (blood thinner). The dose for adults in one study was 100 mg two times a day in adults. As noted above, 100 mg a day in children is useful in migraine prevention.

12. Chronic Venous Insufficiency (CVI) improves with walking, aquatic exercise, elastic stocking and pycnogenol (360 mg). Pycnogenol was more effective than horse chestnut seed extract (600 mg daily) which is known to help with CVI.

13. Back Pain is the fifth most common reason for all physician visits. Ninety percent of adults experience back pain in their life. Fifty percent of the working population complains of back pain annually. Medical management includes NSAIDS (non-steroidal anti-inflammatory drug), physical therapy, epidural steroid injections, and surgery. Studies are divided on the usefulness of acupuncture; however, it is recommended for some patients. Many studies show positive results. (I can tell you acupuncture works! Pilates helps as well. I, personally, have had better results from alternative approaches.)

14. Green Tea. There is growing data to support the anti-tumor properties of green tea. It is used to prevent breast and prostate cancer and should be considered. Take three cups per day or 400 mg of standardized extract. Green tea extract in ointment or capsule form can be a potential therapy regimen for patients with HPV (human papilloma virus) infected cervical lesions. Take 200 mg per day.

15. Butterbur is a member of the daisy family. It inhibits the release of histamine, so it helps in allergic rhinitis. Petaforce and Petadolex are trade names. DO NOT TAKE it in its raw unprocessed form, as it is toxic. The dose in adults is as follows:
    Petaforce 25-50 mg, two to three times per day.
    Petadolex 25-75 mg, two to three times per day
    Tesalin, one to two tabs, two to three times per day.
    Children ten to twelve years old can take 50 mg once daily.
    Do not take if you are pregnant.

16. Insomnia is found in 30 to 35 percent of Americans. Ten percent is chronic (lasting greater than six months). It is the most common sleep complaint to patients' physicians. Sleep quality is inadequate or non-restorative despite adequate opportunity to sleep. Problems include difficulty falling asleep, sleep easily disrupted by multiple spontaneous waking, or early morning waking with the inability to fall back asleep.

    Insomnia usually results from a combination of biologic, physical, psychological, and environmental factors. It is linked with significant morbidity and mortality (Insomnia doubles the risk for fatigue related motor vehicle accidents). In Chinese medicine, insomnia is an underlying Qi imbalance—an imbalance of the mind and its different mental aspects. Acupuncture studies show significant improvement in insomnia with acupuncture treatment, and it should be considered as part of an initial intervention.

17. Probiotics (beneficial bacteria in the colon) re-inoculate and normalize unbalanced normal micro flora in the gut. A few specific probiotics strains have been studied and have shown benefit. These friendly microorganisms have been shown to improve microbial balance in the intestinal tract and display both antibacterial and immune regulatory effects in humans.

    The overly hygienic environment in which most children in developed countries live lacks microbial stimulation, and this may result in an impaired gut barrier that may in turn cause autoimmune, infectious, and inflammatory conditions. (Said simply, being too clean can lead to disease.) This situation may also be associated with IBS (Irritable Bowel Syndrome), IBD (Inflammatory Bowel Disease), and AAD (antibiotic associated diarrhea).

Lactobacillus GG for Clostridium difficile diarrhea has positive results. It also helps prevent relapses of C. difficile in children. Lactobacillus strains that are good for interventions include *L. acidophilus, L. bulgaris, Lactobacillus GG, and L. reuteri.* (The "L" is lactobacillus in all the names listed.) They help reduce the duration of acute infectious diarrhea by approximately one day. In infants, *Bifidobacterium bifidum* helps prevent nosocomial (acquired in the hospital) diarrhea.

Lactobacillus GG has the potential to increase gut IgA immune response and promote the gut immunological barrier. One study reported a significant improvement in Crohn's disease after taking this probiotic.

C. difficile overgrowth has become known as the agent most associated with AAD. It occurs in 3 to 39 percent of patients between initiation of antibiotic treatment and up to two months after the end of treatment. The incidence of diarrhea is 20 to 40 percent in kids on broad-spectrum antibiotics.

Lactobacillus GG is well researched and has a proven safety profile. It is resistant to stomach and bile acids and has the ability to temporarily colonize human intestines. Two studies show that ten to twenty billion CFUs (colony forming units) of LGG/ day significantly decrease the incidence of diarrhea in children.

Supplemental forms of probiotics provide a substantially higher dose of probiotics and appear to be more effective than fermented foods in treating GI disorders.

Do not use large doses of probiotics in patients with severe debilitating illness or altered immune function.

18. Calcium
   ♥ The most abundant mineral in the human body
   ♥ Ninety-nine percent is stored in the skeletal system.

♥ Foods high in calcium include sardines, dairy (especially ricotta cheese, yogurt, and milk), tofu, sesame seeds, collards, and soybeans.

♥ Absorption is variable depending on what is ingested (25 to 50 percent is absorbed, and absorption varies by age). As we age, we develop less stomach HCL (achlorhydria). Infants have the highest absorption rates at 60 percent and young adults at 25 percent. Absorption occurs in the duodenum and proximal jejunum.

♥ Caffeine decreases intestinal absorption when calcium intake is 800 mg per day and increases renal excretion.

♥ Diets high in protein or sodium increase urinary excretion.

♥ Calcium citrate and calcium carbonate are equally absorbed in patients with normal gastric acid. In those with achlorhydria, (no acid secretion in the gut) calcium citrate is better absorbed. Calcium carbonate is better absorbed when taken with a meal.

♥ Postmenopausal women—calcium citrate is better because it prevents bone resorbtion. Coral calcium may contain unsafe levels of lead and mercury.

♥ Calcium can interfere with the absorption of iron, zinc, biophosphonates, tetracycline, quinolones (antibiotics like Cipro, Levaquin, Avalox), and levothyroxine (thyroid replacement). It should be taken separately from medications.

♥ Recommended daily intake for age groups:

Zero to six months	210 mg/d
Seven to twelve months	270 mg/d
One to three years	500mg/d
Four to eight years	800 mg/d
Nine to eighteen years	1300 mg/d
Nineteen to fifty years	1000 mg/d
Fifty-one years+	1200 mg/d

19. Vitamin C and heart disease in women—Vitamin C is necessary for the synthesis of collagen. As an antioxidant, it protects LDL cholesterol from oxidative damage. Lipoprotein-A is decreased in the presence of vitamin C. Frequent aspirin use can decrease vitamin C levels; 250-1000 mg per day of vitamin C can help decrease coronary heart disease (CHD). Risk factor modification has been shown to decrease heart disease risk by 82 percent. Vitamin C is found in citrus fruits, strawberries, cantaloupe, tomatoes, cabbage, broccoli, and dark leafy vegetables.

20. St. John's Wort increases the rate of breakthrough bleeding and potentially affects the metabolism of oral contraceptives (i.e., it increases metabolism and makes them less effective). Its best use so far is in the treatment of mild depression.

21. Ginger is helpful with nausea and vomiting during pregnancy. The preferred method of treatment is capsules. The dose of dried ginger is 1g in three to four divided daily doses. It can also be a digestive aid. It is considered a warm to hot natured food so do not take if spicy foods trigger migraines.

22. PMS is the cyclic occurrence of symptoms that are of sufficient severity to interfere with some aspects of life and that appear with consistent and predictable relationship to menses. No one etiology has been found for PMS.
    Treatments include:
    ♣ Mind-body approach.
    ♣ Aerobic exercise.
    ♣ Supplementation with vitamins, minerals and complex carbohydrates.
    ♣ SSRIs (selective serotonin reuptake inhibitors), OCPs (oral contraceptive pills), and anxiolytics (meds that help with anxiety).
    ♣ Calcium 1200-1600 mg per day will replete the underlying deficiency.
    ♣ Magnesium 200 mg per day can decrease fluid retention.

23. Glucosamine Sulfate is the first structure modifying treatment for knee osteoarthritis, and is greater with mild osteoarthritis

than more advanced disease. Bromelain may also help decrease symptoms of osteoarthritis and rheumatoid arthritis. Dose is 200-400mg per day of Bromelain. Acupuncture can also reduce symptoms.

24. Acupuncture is effective in treating and/or preventing tension or migraine headaches and is a viable option in their treatment.

25. Cervical Cancer is diagnosed worldwide with 500,000 cases per year. Invasive cervical cancer is more common in middle-aged and older women of poor socioeconomic status. The cause of cervical cancer is unknown, but HPV is found in 80 percent of cervical cancer. Smokers have a twofold increase risk to develop cervical cancer. Vegetable consumption and circulating cis-lycopene may be protective against HPV persistence. Condoms prevent most STDs, including HPV.

26. Acupuncture can help treat mild to moderate anxiety and depression especially in those who have had an adverse reaction to medication.

27. Peppermint oil reduces gastric motility by directly acting on gut calcium channels to relax gastrointestinal smooth muscle (by relaxing the smooth muscles in the walls of the intestine, it decreases rapid emptying and irritability of the stomach and intestines). It relaxes the lower esophageal sphincter (so it is contraindicated in GERD—gastro esophageal reflux disease, gallbladder problems, and pregnancy). The primary essential extract is menthol. Use enteric coated preparations. The daily dose is 0.6 ml peppermint oil in capsules or tabs (0.2 ml three times a day before food).

28. Acupuncture has a positive therapeutic affect on osteoarthritis of the knees.

29. Anxiety increases hot flashes in women. That is why Zoloft and Paxil are so successful. It is worse in the later stages of menopause and in African Americans. Hormone levels are NOT associated with anxiety but positively associated with hot flashes (duh). Relaxation techniques have been shown to help a lot!

30. Flaxseed oil (25 grams a day) can help decrease total cholesterol, decrease LDL (bad cholesterol) and prevent breast cancer in postmenopausal women.

The following are interesting medical tidbits gathered from pediatric medical literature.

1. Among patients four to eighteen years old presenting with chief complaint of headaches, symptoms that may indicate the presence of a brain tumor or stroke include vomiting, an abnormal neurological examination, and NO family history of migraine.

2. Children experiencing toilet training difficulties are more likely to be less adaptable and more negative in mood when compared with children who are fully toilet trained.

3. The risk of atopic dermatitis (eczema) at eighteen months increases with each episode of infectious disease in the first six months of life.

4. Children under the age of one who receive antibiotics have an increased risk of developing asthma by age seven.

5. Serial measurements of height and weight indicate that crossing two major percentile lines is most common for children zero to six months and least common for children twenty-four to sixty months.

6. Breath holding spells in childhood have been shown to be associated with syncopal (fainting) episodes later in life.

7. Recurrent abdominal pain in children has been associated with irregular meal patterns, frequent consumption of ice cream and soft drinks, and infrequent eating of fruits and vegetables.

8. In patients with celiac disease, migraine and non-specific headaches improve markedly on a gluten free diet (Wheat free). Gluten is the stuff that makes

grains sticky. It is found in wheat, oats, and barley. Millet, buckwheat, and amaranth are usually fine.

9. Among adolescents, viewing television for more than three hours per day is associated with an increased risk of sleep problems.

10. Prompt myringotomy (incision and drainage of the ear drum) with tube insertion for young children with persistent middle ear effusions is associated with greater prevalence of tympanosclerosis (scarring of the eardrum), retraction pockets, perforation, and cholesteatoma (a fatty tumor) at age five years when compared with late treatment (waiting six months or more with effusion).

11. When compared with children in general, obese children are much more likely to be affected by constipation and/or fecal soiling than non-obese children are.

12. State laws mandating child access protection laws for firearms have been associated with an 8.3 percent reduction in suicide rates among fourteen- to seventeen-year-olds. This is statistically significant.

13. Pediatric-onset of Crohn's disease is most likely to be diagnosed after eight years old and greatest after thirteen years old. It might be associated with Mycobacterium avium; subspecies paratuberculosis.

14. Up to 50 percent of children with celiac disease are completely asymptomatic. They can present with short stature alone.

15. Varicella (chicken pox) vaccination reduces the secondary attack rate among children exposed to unvaccinated cases from approximately 70 percent to 15 percent. (I find this interesting. It does not change my view on the vaccine).

16. Daily persistent headaches in children are most often characterized as unilateral (one sided), pressing or

tightening, and of mild to moderate intensity. Its cause is unknown.

17. Nasal inhalation of aqueous beclomethasone (nasal steroids) has proven effective in controlling BOTH allergic rhinitis and asthma in children five to seventeen years old.

18. Sleep deprivation has not been shown to increase the likelihood of detecting epileptiform (seizure) discharges on EEG obtained in children.

19. Premature birth (less than twenty-eight weeks or less than 1000 gm birth weight) is associated with a significant increase in the occurrence of asthma, pneumonia, and hospitalization for respiratory illness in childhood.

20. A single oral dose of dexamethasone (0.6 mg/kg) (steroid) has been shown to reduce the severity and duration of croup symptoms in children under six years old.

21. Infants who develop TTN (Transient Tachypnea of the Newborn) or those who have respiratory distress syndrome in the newborn period have an increased risk of asthma later.

22. Patients receiving Rocephin can develop nephrolithiasis (kidney stones) unrelated to gender, dose, duration of treatment, or route of administration. Most cases resolve spontaneously.

23. Healthy young infants cry an average of two to three hours a day.

24. Oral rehydration therapy is as effective as IV fluids for rehydration in moderately dehydrated infants and children. It is more tedious but just as effective.

25. Acute hemorrhagic cystitis (grossly bloody urinary tract infection) is commonly caused by adenovirus serotypes eleven and twenty-one.

26. The factor most strongly associated with an infant not sleeping six to nine consecutive hours at night

at nine months of age is feeding the child after an awakening.

27. The severity of an RSV (respiratory syncytial virus) infection may have a genetic basis.

28. Pediatric melanoma is estimated to account for 1 to 3 percent of all childhood neoplasms (cancers). It is estimated that by 2010, one in fifty Americans will develop melanoma at some point in their lives.

29. Newborns continue to amaze us. Newborns are able to recognize their mother's voice and the smell of her breast milk. Infants showed enhanced brain activity while hearing mother's voice compared to that of strangers. Another study showed that exposing newborns to maternal odors calmed them and reduced pain responses during heel sticks.

30. Reading to children and telling stories increases their language development. For each hour of DVD/ video viewing per day, there is a decrease in language development. Current recommendations are no media viewing under age two and no more than one hour a day thereafter.

Chapter Five

Making the Most of Your Visit With the Doctor

Medicine is an art backed by science. Have you ever noticed it is called the "practice of medicine?" Medicine is not a defined science like math with specific and never changing answers to problems. People are the same, but their problems and illnesses are not. Many variables affect us and how we respond to illness and health. Fortunately, research and experience cause medicine to change on a daily basis.

DNA was discovered in 1941. Penicillin was discovered in 1928 and manufactured as an antibiotic in 1941, and was first used at the end of WWII. Now look at how many antibiotics are available and the resultant problems we have with developing resistant strains of bacteria. This has developed in just over sixty years! Think about what else has changed in sixty years.

I have been in practice for twenty-three years. Much of what I learned in medical school is obsolete today. It is IMPOSSIBLE for any physician today to keep abreast of all the changes that happen every day. Each specialty in medicine uses distinct categories of pharmaceutical medicines that do not always apply to other specialties. Categories of medications used by the infectious disease specialists will differ from the commonly used medications of the kidney or gastrointestinal specialists. Most of the medicines we use in pediatrics are used by adults but not vice versa. Adult medicine uses whole classes of medications that we never use in pediatrics because they are unsafe in children. Therefore, pediatricians are truly unable to keep up with the world of adult medicine because it is not our field of practice.

Trauma has changed the most. Today we can now save lives after trauma that fifty years ago were certain to be lost. Because of what we learned in the fields in Vietnam in MASH (Mobile Army Surgical Hospital) units, trauma triage treatment and surgery has advanced a great deal. New changes are occurring because of the war in Iraq. More soldiers' lives are saved every day because of new technology and improved trauma care at the point of injury (in the field where the injury occurred). We also know that lifestyle (smoking, drinking, not wearing seat belts, high blood pressure, and genetics) affects the lives of people in ways medicine cannot fix! It is crucial to remember that you are in charge of your own health.

The word "physician" comes from the Greek root *"physis"* which means *harmony.* We attempt to help you *restore* your body to *harmony* and smooth functioning. By definition, the patient has a central role in this process. When the patient is noncompliant or unwilling to be part of the healing process, the physician cannot help. When patients do not get well, they often blame the doctor. When a physician offers a course of therapy that the patient does not follow, the patient is accountable; not the physician.

When you go to the doctor, it is because you need help. You, the patient, expect the physician to have experience and wisdom. The physician gives you the best he or she has available at that moment. Sometimes it is glorious, and sometimes it is not. We, as physicians, are limited by what you, the patient, tell us (in terms of history) how extensive the disease process is, and by what medicines are available to treat the problem. Likewise, we expect you to give us your best. We expect you to be honest and truthful by telling us all that is going on. If you watch *House* on TV, you will see that many adult patients do not disclose all that is important to their case. Fortunately, pediatrics does not have this same issue.

Primary Care Physicians

There is no shortage of bad publicity about doctors these days. There is also a lot that is still good. I thought it would be a good idea to give you some insight into the nuts and bolts of everyday life in a physician's practice (okay, my practice).

Primary care physicians are the frontline of medicine. We are the grunts, the infantry, and the foot soldiers. We see all the common problems and the really complex ones as well. We do not do a lot of fancy procedures. We do not do surgery.

I feel it is important to clarify the myth that all doctors are rich. This simply is not true. We receive payment based on the face-to-face time we have with patients as we listen, examine, and analyze information to get to the root of the problem. Our reimbursement is no match for more procedure-oriented medicine. Payment for testing goes to the testers.

There is always "chart work to do." There are telephone calls to be addressed, and follow-up questions from patients that need to be answered. It takes several hours a day just to get through the paperwork in order to provide quality care for patients.

Hours

Most medical practices are open Monday through Friday, although some larger practices have evening and Saturday hours. My practice is open Monday through Friday. We see patients from 8:30 a.m. to 4:30 p.m. We do not work evenings or weekends so we can have quality time with our children. All the providers with whom I work are dedicated to their families as well as to our patients. We each work different hours to accommodate work and family.

Appointments

Some practices have "walk-in" appointments. Our practice does not encourage walk-ins. We do encourage patients to make an appointment, and that time is reserved for you and your child to discuss your concerns for that visit.

Patients are scheduled in fifteen to thirty minute blocks. It takes TIME to talk to someone and determine what is going on, along with the best way to handle the situation at the time. An uncomplicated visit can be done in fifteen minutes. More complex or involved cases require thirty minutes or more. The appointment time is the *actual* time that a patient should be in the room with a physician. If a patient shows up late, then the providers run late the rest of the day. Patients need to arrive fifteen minutes BEFORE their appointment time so the nursing personnel can get their vital signs, and get them checked in and ready for the healthcare provider. Sometimes patients have more medical problems than expected, or a patient is much sicker than expected, and needs more time and treatment than anticipated. These unplanned complications can cause the healthcare provider to fall behind schedule.

When you are lucky to have an early morning appointment, it is extremely important, and advantageous, to arrive early. In the morning, you can be in and out quickly. If you are late for the first appointment of the day, everyone after you must wait.

Our schedules are not overbooked. We can see a maximum of twenty patients per provider in a full day. We do not believe in seeing more patients than we can comfortably evaluate and for whom we can provide quality care. Each patient receives what he or she needs in a visit, and questions are answered. This practice is busy, and our philosophy is to provide quality care.

We appreciate it when patients wait, and we do apologize for the wait. It's most likely that someone ahead of you really needed help. It is always possible to reschedule your appointment if your schedule is too tight. (I have done that several times personally). I appreciate the help and care I get from my doctors. If they are tied up and my schedule is tight, I reschedule. Is it inconvenient? Yes, but I want the best from my physician and from me, and that cannot happen if one of us is super stressed and the other does not understand.

Everyone gets stressed. It is especially hard to wait for a long time with a sick or active child. Please know we appreciate your frustration and we do our best. We know how the frustration can lead to a sour mood, sarcasm, or just feeling rude. Please count to ten or decompress since being rude accomplishes nothing.

We do our best to understand that patients have schedules, too, but illness is not a simple consumer product. Illness is individual, and different people require different treatments. Not every visit can be done in five minutes and every concern resolved. As healthcare providers, we really dislike being behind in our schedules, and we really do not like patients to wait. However, the providers with whom I work have integrity and caring hearts, and are willing to give each patient what he or she needs at the time, even if it means going a bit over on the time.

Many patients have asked if they can come late because the doctor is running late. This is a good question, and one I pondered for years. I finally realized that waiting at the doctor's office is like being in line at Disney. If you leave the line, no one will hold your spot! Everyone wants a turn as much as you do. We apologize when you have to wait. You still must arrive on time for your appointment.

Insurance and Payment

Since medical practices are "insurance based," it is essential to have current and correct information for filing patient claims timely and efficiently. Claims are filed electronically these days, which means turnaround time is weeks instead of months.

Until the electronic medical record is inexpensive and streamlined, many practices will continue to have paper records. We certainly do. On January 1 of each year, new insurance cards are issued. Many families change addresses, insurance companies, schools, or phone numbers. Therefore, it is crucial to fill out new forms at the beginning of each year. Is it a tedious pain to fill out new information every year? YES. Many parents do not like filling out the forms. It serves no purpose to be angry about circumstances beyond your control and ours. AGAIN, without your correct and CURRENT information, insurance cannot be filed correctly and the claim will be rejected. This will result in your having to pay for the visit out of pocket. We really stress that providing correct insurance information is your responsibility. You can now download the registration form and assignment of benefits forms from our web site so the forms can be filled out before you come into the office. I hope that this will reduce some of your stress. The website is www.franzcenter.com. Many offices now have their forms on their web sites.

Most insurance claims are paid within thirty days because of the efficiency of electronic billing. In my practice, any claim that has not been paid by 120 days after the claim is filed becomes the patient's out-of-pocket responsibility.

Physicians practice medicine because they love helping people. It is a business with many expenses. It is HOW we, and our staff, make a living. I cannot imagine any other business person not expecting to be paid for his or her services.

How can you help in receiving the best care?

Many patients do not have insurance. That is a choice that the patient makes, or it may be as simple as not being able to get or afford insurance. It is important to let your doctor's office know if you do not have insurance. Many offices do offer a cash discount.

We do our best to keep costs down, and we understand the challenges and difficulties of medical care costs. We will not jeopardize the health of your loved one by not ordering necessary testing. Healthcare is expensive, and there are times that X-rays, MRI, or CTs (CAT scan) are needed and cannot be avoided. It is unfair to you, your family, and your healthcare provider to think that there are shortcuts. There are not.

Make the most of your face-to-face time with your doctor by knowing the following.

1. If you have multiple problems or physical complaints, you may require more than one visit to address them properly. A long list of multiple body system problems or complaints cannot effectively be addressed and treated in a short office visit.
2. Write out your questions before your office visit.
3. If you have a lot of questions, it can help to send them via e-mail or fax a day or two before the visit. This gives the health care provider time to consider them, look up anything if necessary, and let you know what

can be handled in the upcoming visit and what items might require an additional visit.

4. Well-visits are now a time to discuss wellness and prevention strategies. Most practices, including ours, do not discuss illness issues, behavior problems, or chronic problems at a well visit. A separate visit is needed for non-well issues.

5. If your healthcare provider needs to order labs, get them done as soon as possible. It is not in your best interest to procrastinate.

6. It is our office policy to collect your co-pay (please know what it is!) upon arrival and check in, BEFORE you see your healthcare provider. Some practices collect it at the end of the visit.

7. Practices appreciate constructive feedback. If someone in the office is rude to you or there is a problem, let the office manager know. No system is perfect, and no system can make improvements without constructive feedback. Problems cannot be fixed if no one hears about them.

8. Know your pharmacy number and have it available. This makes a BIG difference when prescriptions need to be called in or faxed to the pharmacy.

9. If a parent or spouse cannot accompany you at the visit, send a list of questions. It is not appropriate to have someone bring in the patient and then expect the healthcare provider to call the one who could not make it to explain the visit all over again. It is not possible.

10. Please refrain from asking about a child who is not present. The scheduled appointment time is for the patient who is present.

11. I personally have a big issue with patients being rude to the staff. Unnecessary rudeness (which is a funny statement because I do not think there is a time of necessary rudeness) can get you dismissed from the

practice. Sometimes staff members are only doing what they were told to do. If you are having trouble communicating with the staff, then ask for the office manager. There is usually a reasonable way to resolve your differences and concerns without being rude.

Medicine is a business now because of the explosion of illness, changes in what we know, and volume of people that need to be seen. One hundred years ago an accident in the field meant death. Now a team of people can save that person, and as you are aware, there are thousands of accidents every day! Many physicians now work in shifts, which enables us to provide optimal care.

When I started my practice, I had no rules. I believed in kindness, courtesy, and in doing the right thing for the right reason. As you can guess, not everyone holds those same values. Now I have rules to help keep you and my practice safe. I also have rules so that the days flow smoothly, and we can meet the needs of as many people as possible.

Communication with the Doctor

There is only one gold standard for communicating with the physician. This is a face- to-face visit. Most offices still have some form of phone communication. However, true phone communication should be confined to getting lab results and making appointments. Most offices no longer call in prescriptions. Patients need to make an appointment to be seen. This is a crucial change in the last ten years and important for patients to understand. Litigation over minor issues has created an environment where physicians cannot assume responsibility for a patient or patient's condition if the patient has not been seen in the office. It is inappropriate to ask the doctor to call in a medicine without seeing the patient. This places the physician and the patient at risk.

The second best way to communicate directly with your doctor is through a fax message. The fax is the written word and becomes part of the medical record. You can be specific and detailed, which helps the doctor. The faxed message is generally answered directly by a healthcare provider.

I also love e-mail for basic questions and general information. E-mail is not the forum for intimate or private information since the Internet is not secure. That is why the fax or face-to-face visit is better.

Understand the policies for answering phone calls, and e-mails, etc. Physicians deal with patients who are in the office first. Phone calls are often answered in a day or two. Most e-mails and faxes are addressed in some fashion the same day or within twenty-four hours.

After Hours

All practices have someone on call after hours. Our practice uses Telekids. Telekids is staffed by RNs (registered nurses) with pediatric experience. They have set written protocols that are faxed to our office the next morning. We know who called, with whom the patient spoke, what the problem was, and what was advised. Our practice charges for this service. There is a fee for speaking with the nurse on call and a separate fee if it is necessary to speak with the MD or ARNP on call.

After-hours calls are for problems that truly cannot wait until the office reopens. After hours are not for requesting refills for medications that you forgot to call about during office hours, nor for minor problems. We are happy to be there for you if you are in need. In our community, we are lucky enough to have two groups who are open after hours. It is also for those times when a child needs to be seen but does not have an emergency. Physicians in hospitals that routinely deliver pediatric care best handle emergency visits. We are fortunate to have the Arnold Palmer Hospital Emergency Department in Orlando.

Regular Visits

Children need regularly scheduled checkups at two months, four months, six months, nine months, twelve months, fifteen months, eighteen months, twenty-four months, and once a year after age two (twenty-four months). I have always found it interesting that the regular checkups are on the same schedule as the immunizations.

Please let us know if you need HRS and/or physical forms for school PRIOR to the visit. We have so many forms to fill out every year that we need advance notice. Summer is the busiest time for well visits and school forms. It takes awhile to fill them out and can cause us to get behind if we do not know about them until the end of the visit. If we are unable to fill out the form on the day of the visit, we will get them completed within twenty-four to forty-eight hours. Due to the huge volume of forms and the rise in postage, we no longer mail forms to parents unless you have provided us with a stamped, self-addressed envelope.

Adolescents need yearly checkups as well. There is much preventive and educational information that we cover, so it is important they keep these appointments. I have found my adolescent sons listen to people other than me, so I relish these appointments! Adolescents tend to begin to form adult habits during these years, and if they neglect their healthcare now, they will neglect it as adults and increase their risk for all kinds of health-related problems.

Choosing a Physician

In many practices, patients see only one doctor. In others, they never see the same person twice. My practice is small, with five total providers. We try to accommodate you by having you see the healthcare provider of your choice. There are times, however, where you need to see the first available provider. This minimizes your wait time and gets your child, especially a sick one, taken care of as soon as possible.

I only work mornings, so afternoon appointments are not available with me. We also request and encourage that you make well appointments with each provider so you get to know them in a non-stressful time; i.e., when your child is NOT sick.

Knowing all the providers in my practice offers great continuity of care for your child. You can see one provider often. However, it is not wise or practical to see only one provider all the time. I am unable to be the only physician all my patients see. It is not feasible when working the hours I work. I hire providers I trust and believe will offer the same quality of care that I offer to patients.

In any practice, you will find providers with whom you really connect, and some with whom you will not. Remember that this is a relationship between doctor and patient, and if you are not happy with the information given, it is important to speak up. We need to be able to see your points and provide care that suits us both. If you are not going to do what the doctor says because you disagree, we both lose, and the patient suffers. There are rare times when I explain to patients that things must be done my way, and with no questions asked. These times generally occur when a patient is really sick, and there is little room for discussion because the patient's life can be affected.

Office Manager

The office manager is an important and key person in every practice! The office manager helps resolve communication issues, billing problems, staff issues, and other problems you may encounter. The providers are generally busy taking care of patients and cannot handle complaints in an effective manner. It is good to know the office manager! The manager knows the day-to-day operation issues better than the providers.

Hospital Affiliations

At what hospitals does your doctor have privileges? Does your doctor see patients in the hospital, and if so, when does he or she make rounds? Nationwide, hospitalists are now seeing the patients in the hospital. Hospitalists are board certified physicians who practice only in the hospital setting and then release the patient back to his or her primary care physician. My practice uses hospitalists who are colleagues of mine, and whom I trust implicitly. They make rounds several times a day and provide excellent in-house care. They also see all my newborns.

Our practice affiliation is with only one hospital system—Arnold Palmer Hospital for Children and the new Winnie Palmer Hospital for Babies and Women.

Again, knowing your insurance coverage and benefits is crucial. If your insurance affiliated hospital is Florida Hospital, we need to know. Admission there is provided by a different group of hospitalists who are also wonderful.

It is also important that you know what laboratory serves your insurance. If you get labs done at a non-participating lab, you have to pay the cost out of pocket. Generally we know, but two heads are better than one!

Alternative Medicine

When my oldest was three years old, he became very sick, and all that I knew in traditional medicine was not helping. I ventured into the world of alternative medicine, and was deeply rewarded. I went back to school to learn about homeopathy and have ever since incorporated alternative medicine tools and testing into my practice. We like trying to find the root cause (we don't always succeed, but we do make major progress). There are many avenues of alternative medicine available; I have chosen only a handful to use. This practice offers homeopathy and Chinese herbs. We have a list of other excellent alternative-based practitioners whom we can recommend.

There are additional fees for these services, as they are not the "standard" traditional medical therapies. I love having a choice for patients so that traditional medications are not always the only answer!

We thank you for entrusting the care of your family to us. We do our best to keep you happy (and us—a happy doctor provides good care!) As we grow or encounter experiences that necessitate change, you will see new "rules." We do our best to keep you informed.

The following list of manners was created due to a violation of these manners. Children view the world as a playground, and it is our job as adults and parents to teach and guide them to be respectful of other people's belongings.

It is never too early to teach your children manners, values, and safety. Please observe the following when you are here:

1. The rolling stool belongs to the doctor and nurse practitioner. Please do not play on it, eat on it, or use it as a storage unit.

2. While we use washable paint on the walls, we have found it difficult to get many marks off the walls. Please do not put your feet all over the walls. Please do not draw on them or throw toys that could damage the walls.

3. Please do not make stray marks on the exam tables. If your child needs to draw, please have a book or something firm to back it, so the table is not marred.

4. We choose not to lock our one cabinet in the exam room. Please do not let your children play with or in the cabinets as they could get injured or damage our property.

5. One lesson I have learned is never to play with or borrow anything that you cannot afford or do not wish to replace. The ear and eye looker light (otoscope/opthalmoscope) is very expensive.

6. The massage tables that we use have knobs on the legs, so we can adjust the height. The knobs are appealing to small children, but the table will fall if they remove the knobs.

7. While we are a pediatric office and do cater to children, it is still a medical office and <u>not</u> a playground. It is helpful for children to learn how to behave respectfully in our facility.

Thank you very much.

Chapter Six

A Nontraditional Approach to the Chronically Ill Child

There are two kinds of chronically ill children—those with an actual chronic disease, usually with a genetic basis, (cystic fibrosis, Sickle Cell Disease, tumors, etc.), and those who are healthy but recurrently sick. This information deals with the latter.

Many children who start day care will experience a time of recurrent illnesses simply because the child is exposed to more illnesses. We call this "exercising the immune system" and it is a good thing when the child recovers within a few days and does not need repeated doctor visits and medications. The ones that concern me are those who end up on recurrent antibiotics.

When I see such a child for the first time, it is most important to obtain a good history. Some children have a genetic predisposition that makes them more susceptible to getting sick. Hence, a good family history is important. What illnesses are there in the family tree regarding parents, grandparents, aunts, uncles, cousins, and three generations back?. Please do not make excuses like, "He had cancer because he smoked." Cancer is cancer and is in the family tree regardless of how he got it. Not every smoker gets cancer and not every cancer patient smokes.

Other children have non-genetic issues that can be addressed, and thus reduce susceptibility to illness.

The first question is about labor and delivery. Prolonged labor, difficult labor, or precipitous delivery can all affect the baby in a long-term way. Babies born with *cone heads* had a long duration in the birth canal, and the subsequent molding of the head at birth can strain the underlying tissues and result in increased susceptibility to sinus infections and/or ear infections. Premature babies have their own class of susceptibilities.

Next, I am interested in the health of the child in specific time increments. How was the health of the child from birth to six months? Six months to a year? Twelve months to eighteen months, etc.? This allows us to see if there was a specific incident, illness, or point in time that the child became ill and has essentially "never been well since."

Did this child have vaccines? How many at a time? Were there any reactions to the shots? Was there a point in time where the child's health seemed to get worse after vaccines? Sometimes I hear that after every vaccine the child got a bad cold, but recovered after a few weeks. I am looking for trends in health patterns.

Next, we do a physical exam. Usually the patient looks great, and there is no evidence of illness on the initial visit. Such a healthy exam is always a good sign and does not negate the history that we just elicited.

There are three basic levels in the body where illness can occur, and then be addressed for restoring balance—mechanical, chemical, and energetic.

Mechanical therapy addresses physical problems in the actual structure or mechanics of the musculoskeletal system. Massage, chiropractic, Rolfing, etc. are therapies that help in this area.

Chemical therapy is accomplished with medicines, herbs, supplements, vitamins, foods, and anything that nourishes the chemical environment of the body. This environment deals with the metabolic imbalances, toxins, hormones, bacteria, etc. in the body.

Energetic therapy includes Reiki, acupuncture, healing touch, homeopathy, Chinese herbs, prayer, and other modalities that deal with the energetic plane of the body. This is the non-physical area of the body. We do know it exists. Therapies here are definitely more mind-oriented and help the body. All dis-harmony begins in the energetic body. When the energetic part of the being is disturbed, the issue must be addressed. It then will manifest in physical or mental symptoms, and the organism begins to restore harmony.

Having a good history to see where obstacles might lie helps determine how to proceed.

Determining how much dairy a patient consumes is very important. Simply eliminating milk from the diet can have a profound healing effect on many children. Some do well just stopping liquid milk, and others must eliminate all dairy products—cheese, yogurt, butter, sour cream, cream cheese, and cottage cheese, for a time. Dairy can be very allergenic at a subacute level; meaning it does not have immediate reactions like hives, sneezing, diarrhea, etc., but can have delayed reactions that show up as eczema, chronic runny nose, recurrent ear and sinus infections, and generally feeling ill.

Many children have an imbalance in their intestinal bacteria (flora) balance. There are bacteria in our intestines to digest foods and create an internal healthy environment. This BALANCE is necessary and there is some thought that the proper balance of "good bacteria" actually allows them to make natural antiviral chemicals and fight off illness at the intestinal level. When bacterial balance is lost due to lots of antibiotics or because the infant did not get properly colonized passing through mom's birth canal, then the resulting imbalance can predispose the child to getting ill more easily.

Medicines and shots can deplete the body of natural illness-fighting vitamins. The MMR drains vitamin A stores. Medicines drain many vitamins. Omega three fatty acids can be insufficient from birth and from diet. Our diets really are not great these days. Research shows how important vegetables are. They are natural chelators. (Fruits help regenerate the flesh, and seeds repair DNA, according to Chinese medicine.) They keep us healthy; more so than fruits. They contain antioxidants, fiber, and other essential nutrients. They improve cognition (the latest study shows Alzheimer patients improve with vegetables. How many of us have children who do not like vegetables?).

In general, here are some suggestions I make to begin to improve the child's health. It is also important to have the child seen with each illness after implementing these changes, since the next step to wellness is to get off the antibiotic merry-go-round. Each time a child can get through a minor illness without antibiotics, the immune system gets stronger. Nature does a better job than we do 90 percent of the time. If medicine is necessary, it will be prescribed. I will not endanger the health of the child while we improve his/her immune system, but each time we have to use antibiotics, beneficial bacteria are being killed as well as the bad bacteria. Recognizing the effects of each treatment modality is important. Actions can be taken to minimize the side effects of antibiotics when they are necessary.

1. Stop milk.
2. Begin probiotics (good BACTERIA). Children under seven use Bifidophilus one-half to one teaspoon two times a day. Infants use one-eighth teaspoon twice a day, for a minimum of six months, and then we can reevaluate. Probiotic treatment may continue indefinitely.
3. Children over seven years can take the mixed flora with acidophilus, lactobacillus, etc.
4. Children over two months of age can begin supplementation with "good yeast" (Saccharomyces boulardii) called Florastor. The dose is the same for all people two months and up. The good yeast in the gut secretes a sugar coating that attracts the bad yeast and bacteria and then they are pooped out. I recommend the Florastor for two to three months and then we can reevaluate. Some patients develop diarrhea on probiotics. Stop them if this occurs.
5. Begin omega three fatty acids. DHA Jr is chewable fish oil made by Nordic Naturals. It has a pleasant strawberry taste. For those who are allergic to fish or want a non-animal alternative, try Total Essential Fatty acids, Udo oil, flax seed oil, or Expecta.

6. For those with a history of lots of falls or a difficult birth process, I also recommend a chiropractor AND/ OR Craniosacral therapy (which is a gentle form of adjustment). For those who are concerned about the chiropractor, I have found that chiropractors use gentle pressure in children and not the perceived "snap, crackle, pop" so many of us think happens. I have had many patients respond well to the multilevel treatments. (Using mechanical and chemical levels of therapy.) After all, our goal is improved health. I remind patients that it is possible to treat a broken bone with homeopathic remedies to speed healing, but all the remedies in the world will not set the bone straight if it is displaced. We need mechanical intervention by orthopedics to set the bone in the proper position so the remedies can get it to heal.

7. Make dietary adjustments to include more fruits and vegetables. I also recommend a product called Juice Plus ™, which is fifteen fruits and vegetables and two grains, freeze dried in a gummy or a capsule. It is a WHOLE food supplement and thus contains the total complex of nutrients from those foods, not just single vitamins. It is not meant to replace good eating, but for those stubborn children who don't like to eat veggies, this is a good alternative. When they get the nutrients from the JuicePlus™, they will gradually want to eat the actual foods.

8. There is a test we offer called Spectracell that measures twenty-eight nutrients at the cellular level. It takes three weeks to obtain the test results as the white cells are grown, and as nutrients are added and subtracted to see what nutrient insufficiencies the patient's cells have.

9. I also recommend the Dried Blood Assessment to see what general organ system insufficiencies there might be. Details on this are addressed elsewhere.

With this approach, the patient can begin to take steps to recover good health. The patient will need to take vitamin and herbal supplements, generally in small amounts. The biggest challenge becomes the commitment to getting these in the child. I just remember what the objective is—improved health and fewer doctor visits. If the pattern of illness continues, parents will be giving repeated antibiotics with less and less effectiveness over time. Therefore, it is easier to take supplements that improve health than medicine all the time.

Remember, YOU are the adult. Supplements are given morning and evening to fit the working parents' lifestyle and to minimize having to give something numerous times a day (everyone gets tired of that).

With a good history and physical exam, we can embark on the journey back to health. It does not happen over night. It is process. After all, it took awhile to get to this place of ill health, so it will take awhile to get back.

Simple changes and a few supplements can make dramatic differences if you are willing to make the effort. The longer I am in medicine, the more I see that everyone wants a magic pill to make them better. All the time we hear, "I do not have time for this. I do not have time for my child to be sick. As a physician, I have experienced the same feelings, and it makes me so sad that I can put my child's health second to anything else. I have spent the time to learn these simple techniques, and over time, I have seen my own children's health slowly and steadily improve. There are no shortcuts. There really are no magic pills to make everything better. Generally, symptoms are telling you something about your own body or your child's. So I make the effort to find the root cause. (I do not always find it, but it's not necessary if the changes we make improve health.) The body is an AMAZING organism. Many times when you make one change in one area, there is a domino affect that triggers improvement in other systems. With this, the root cause may take care of itself. Enjoy the journey. It is worth the trip.

Autism

Autism is an evolving field that is constantly changing! At this time, no one knows what causes autism, but we do know now that there is a "brain-gut" connection. It may be there is an autoimmune dysfunction with an underlying genetic predisposition. Some children are born autistic, and for others it seems to be *triggered* by vaccinations (despite what the scientific literature says.) Parents of children with autism will tell you unequivocally that their child was "normal" until fifteen months. After the MMR, they are often clear that their child began to regress. Autism as a naturally occurring disorder (meaning the child was born with it) will manifest between the ages of fifteen- and thirty-six months. The scientific community thinks the shots do not have any bearing, and that it is coincidental with the natural evolution of the disorder.

There are some very interesting facts that are emerging as more and more attention is placed on autism. We know that the incidence has dropped from one in thousands to 1:150. We know that it has increased 800 fold in the last twenty years. We know that retrospective studies claim there is no link between vaccines and autism. In January 2008, the The Orlando Sentinel Orlando Sentinel printed an article starting that researchers believe they have found an "autism gene" on chromosome sixteen. Much work lies ahead to see if this is an important and reproducible finding.

The genetic basis may be a problem with methylation, and hence, heavy metal detoxification. Some kids are born heavy-metal toxic. If their mother worked in a factory, around chemicals, or if they live in certain areas prone to heavy metal problems in the soil and water, the mother may transfer the metals to the fetus via the placenta. There is a gene, the MTHFR (methylenetetrahydofolate reductase), that affects homocysteine metabolism. Homocysteine and methionine are involved in making the antioxidant glutathione. Glutathione helps rid the body of free radicals. Patients who have two copies of this gene, one from the mother and one from the father, are called homozygous positive and will have lifetime issues with homocysteine and glutathione metabolism. The good news is that supplements can be given to prevent problems.

Vitamin B12 is also necessary to make neurotransmitters and for other biochemical reactions in the body. It also helps convert homocysteine to methionine and converts methylmalonic acid to succinic acid. Many autistic children are deficient in methyl B12. There is a simple urine test that can determine this problem. It measures methylmalonic acid (MMA). If the MMA is elevated, there is a deficit of B12. MANY autistic children are deriving significant benefit from MB12 injections and from glutathione supplementation. Methyl B12 is not absorbed well enough in the gut to be able to correct the deficit these patients have. The web site www.drneubrander.com is an excellent resource for methyl B12 information.

For others, the problem with methylation is triggered when given vaccines with Thimerasol.

The MMR vaccine affects vitamin A levels by decreasing them. Vitamin A is also linked to a G-alpha protein, which is connected to retinoid receptors. These two must be linked for speech to occur. When vitamin A levels are drained, the G-alpha protein and the retinoid receptors are disconnected and speech is affected. This symptom presents as a loss of language or as no language development in an affected child. This "disconnect" is why some patients improve when they are given cod liver oil—their vitamin A stores are repleted. By giving vitamin A before and after the MMR vaccine, this can be avoided.

If Thimerasol is the problem (and DAN doctors say it is!) then removing it from vaccines will help. Thimerasol is now removed from all vaccines. Unfortunately, a study in Scandinavia showed that autism rates did not drop when Thimerasol was removed from vaccines. Giving fewer vaccines simultaneously does not overload the immune system and allows the healthcare provider to see which vaccines cause problems. For some patients, the damage can be reversed. For others, it can be too late. Despite our best efforts, the brain cell damage cannot be undone.

There has also been speculation that the measles part of the MMR causes an encephalopathy and a leaky gut. This may or may not be true. There has been positive PCR identification of measles in the spinal fluid and gut; the same DNA as the vaccine.

I view autism, ADD, ADHD, LD (learning disabilities), dyslexia, sensory integration, and giftedness as all on one straight continuum. All these people have similarities in common. Only some have more manifestation of dysfunction than others. Autism is one spot on this continuum.

At one end is the head banging institutionalized autistic child (the image we grew up with) and the other end is the penultimate genius - computer geek, rocket scientist, or inventor. Everything else lies in between—ADD, ADHD, LD, dyslexia, etc. All the autistic kids I have cared for seem to be inherently brilliant; trapped in their own minds. They are not retarded. Studies clearly show that gifted children have a higher chance of having allergies, asthma, and ADD/ADHD. ADD/ADHD is, in my opinion, a much higher functioning version of autism. Their damage is not as great. Also, a gifted teacher once told me that exceptional children run in families. This means that exceptional parents can have a child that is gifted and/or a child with ADD or autism. They are all exceptional. This point is clearly illustrated to me when I look at the children of physicians. Many are very bright and many have reading disabilities, ADD, etc.

Since I believe that vaccines may contribute to triggering autism, I choose to stop vaccines when I see a new patient who is diagnosed with autism. I am unwilling to take the risk that there is a connection. I can give a shot but I cannot undo the damage it does, so why risk it? You cannot un-inject a vaccine.

Obtaining a thorough history is paramount in understanding how and when this child developed symptoms. It will provide clues from family history, pregnancy, labor, and delivery. Vaccination history is also helpful. I will outline questions to which I want answers. This will help you even before you see your physician.

1. How was Mom's health before and when she became pregnant? Does she have any chronic health

problems? Where did she and Dad work? Did either have exposure, ongoing or otherwise to heavy metals? Did either have exposure to chemicals, like working in factories, etc?

2. How was the pregnancy? Any complications? Any stressful events during pregnancy?

3. How was labor? Was it prolonged? When did her membranes rupture? Was the baby term or preterm (earlier than thirty-six weeks)?

4. Was delivery vaginal or by C-section? If C-section, why?

5. Did the baby go home with you after birth at one to two days?

6. Did he or she eat well? Was the baby breast or bottle-fed? Did the baby grow well and gain weight well? Was there jaundice? Did it need treatment? How high was the highest bilirubin?

7. How long did Mom breast-feed? If not, then what formula or formulas were tried and what were the results? Did the baby have problems with cow milk formulas? Soy formulas? Did the baby stool well? Were there any problems with blood in the stool? Constipation?

8. How did the baby grow and develop from birth to two months?

9. Have there been any problems with eczema or allergies?

10. At two months, was everything normal? Did the child receive vaccinations? How many?

11. How did the child grow and develop from two to six months? Did he or she continue to receive vaccinations and how did he or she fare with them?

12. How was growth and development from six to twelve months? Any ear infections? Constipation? Diarrhea? What age did this child walk? Talk?

13. Same for six to eighteen months. Any problems with recurrent infections? Growth? Development? Shots?

14. Eighteen to twenty-four months? Twenty-four to thirty-six months? Thirty-six to forty-eight months, etc.?

15. What specific behavior problems have you noticed and when did they begin? Are there problems with anxiety (separation anxiety)? Flapping of the arms? Aggression?

16. Have you tried removing any foods from the diet? If so, what were the results?

17. Does this child sleep? Has there ever been a sleep problem? If so, when? What have you tried? Did this child have colic? Reflux?

18. If this child has a diagnosis of autism, PDD (Pervasive Developmental Delay), or other, when was he or she diagnosed? Who made the diagnosis?

19. Any problems with seizures? Headaches? Stomach-aches? Vomiting?

20. Anything else you can think to tell us? What therapies have you tried, if any?

There are places in development where we can pick up early concerns for autism. When there are concerns or a sense that something is amiss with your child, early evaluation can be done. My personal approach is to stop or decrease vaccines to one at a time while evaluation is being done. *Vaccines can be given at any time.* However, once they are injected, they cannot be un-injected. Once damage has occurred, it is difficult to reverse. I am VERY conservative when there are any concerns with development. The adage "better safe than sorry" goes a long way with me. Below are some age related developmental concerns (obtained from Autism Magazine, Nov-Dec 2007, p. 9).

At six months
- If a child is not making eye contact with parents during interaction

- If the child is not cooing or babbling (these milestones develop at two and four months)
- If the baby is not making vocal sounds in response to parents (called vocal turn-taking)

At twelve months
- If the child is making no attempt to speak
- If the child is not pointing, waving, or grasping
- If the child is indifferent to others or making no response to his or her name
- If repetitive motions like rocking or hand flapping are observed
- If the child is overly sensitive to smells or sounds
- If there is a loss of language
- If there is strong resistance to change in routine

At twenty-four months
- If there is any loss of language or developmental skill
- If there is no development of language skills
- If there is a gut feeling that "something is not right"

A physical exam is next. Fortunately, there are seldom any physical problems.

After routine labs are drawn and any abnormalities addressed, the following are recommendations that can be tailored to each child. Labs we routinely order include a complete blood count, complete metabolic profile, sedimentation rate, thyroid functions, and tests for celiac disease (antigliadin IgG, TTG or tissue transglutaminase, homocysteine level), and urine test for MMA or methylmalonic acid test to determine if there is a B12 deficiency.

1. First recommendation is a gluten free/casein free diet (GFCF). I recommend they go to www.glutensolutions.com for info. We also recommend a support group for learning to cook GFCF. It takes a

month to clear dairy from the system and up to seven months to clear wheat. It is important to give this diet time to work. If dairy is a major food allergen, its removal will often result in a rapid improvement in speech, and chronic loose stools often substantially improve. There are bakeries springing up that cater to the GFCF lifestyle. Seek them out in your area.

2. The patient needs to be on cod liver oil. Pharmaceutical grade cod liver oil has been processed to remove mercury, and this is what is needed. I recommend DHA jr. or Coromega (a pleasant orange flavored source that comes in "ketchup" like packages). Nordic Naturals and Carlson's are excellent sources of cod liver oil in liquid, chewable, or gel cap form. The new Expecta could be a good source as it is made from algae and hence is mercury free. Expecta is a good source of DHA but not vitamin A. The vitamin A helps the G-alpha protein and retinoid receptors connect. Omega three fatty acids enhance all the cells of the body. Olive oil is an excellent source of omega three, six, and nine fatty acids. I have recently learned from patients that coconut oil has some very beneficial effects on cognitive function.

3. The patient needs a good MVI (multivitamin). I recommend they call Kirkman Labs 1-800-245-8282. Kirkman Labs caters to the autistic patient so everything is GFCF, preservative free, and pleasant tasting, etc. All their products are pharmaceutical grade products. There are many other excellent sources of pharmaceutical grade products.

4. These patients all have leaky gut and intestinal dysbiosis (beneficial bacteria imbalance). All of them will have yeast overgrowth at some point. It is often difficult to get rid of the yeast permanently. It must be treated long term (often four to six months or longer) with low doses of medicine to keep it gone.

I like to test the stool through Genova Diagnostics periodically to see how the patients are doing and to be sure we are using a medication to which the yeast is sensitive. (Great Plains and Doctor Data are companies that also do much of this testing.) I often use Diflucan. Diflucan must be monitored as it can cause liver damage and idiosyncratic decrease in neutrophils in the bone marrow. The herb uva ursi works and so does grapefruit seed extract. Parents will often let me know if something new is around and working on their child. Oregano oil, Pau d'Arco, and other herbs have been known to also safely decrease the yeast overload. ***Do not start these herbs without guidance from a professional.***

5. Autistic patients need to be on probiotics. Culturelle is a popular one as is Pro Bio Gold from Kirkman Labs. Often they need to have several brands and alternate them for better coverage. Threelac™ is another brand that is having good results in some patients. There are many brands that can have a positive effect on the gut.

6. Injections of Vitamin methyl B12 are also recommended for these patients. An excellent web resource for this is www.drneubrander.com. First, the patient needs to have a urine test for MMA.

7. Secretin, IVIG, or IV glutathione are the domain of the autism specialists.

8. Some patients will respond to acyclovir if there is a history of herpes. I have used hair analysis in the past as a screen for heavy metals. It does not reflect total body burden of heavy metals like we thought. I use it on a limited basis now. There is also a urine test for heavy metals. It is two parts through specialty labs like Great Plains, Genova, Doctor Data, and others. The first is a random urine sample that looks at heavy metal excretion in the urine. A single dose of DMSA

(a chelating agent) 10/kg (not more than 200 mg) is given and urine collected for the next six to twelve hours. If there is heavy metal toxicity, there should be a fourfold increase in the excretion. This test is not as reliable as we thought because a lot of the heavy metal burden is in the brain and does not easily come out of the brain with this challenge test.

9. The homeopathic remedy Carcinosin 1M weekly for four weeks is a general remedy for autism. If there is a history of vaccine reactions, I may also recommend Silica 1M weekly for four to eight weeks. I have had some nice results with increased language with this method. *These remedies can be obtained only from a practitioner.*

10. MMR titers (a blood test to measure antibody levels after the vaccine) reflect immunity, and are indicated instead of a second MMR dose.

11. Neuroscience testing is a urine test that reflects epinephrine, norepinephrine, serotonin, GABA, dopamine, glutamate, and phenylethylamine in the urine. Autistic patients often spill glutamine at high rates in the urine and may have other neurotransmitter imbalances that can be helped with supplements. Their web site www.Neuroscienceinc. org is fascinating and informative.

12. Brain mapping with experienced facilities gives a visual map of the brain's executive and cognitive centers, and shows how they are functioning. Therapy is done with neurofeedback to "rewire" the brain and improve function. While it is expensive, it makes a big difference. In the Orlando area, there are three providers who offer neurofeedback services.

13. A lot of patients with autistic spectrum disorder also respond to anti-seizure medicines as prescribed by a neurologist or autism specialist

14. There are genetic tests offered with various companies that will show us if there is a methylation problem. There are two specific loci for methylation that the basic panel shows. Specifically it looks for the MTHFR gene. It is very helpful because it does provide us with genetic information. If methylation metabolism is dysfunctional because it is a DNA issue, then lifelong supplements will be required.

15. Dried Blood Analysis. Please refer to the chapter on this below.

16. Sometimes a Complete Diagnostic Stool Analysis (CDSA) needs to be done (through Genova Diagnostics.) It tells us a lot about digestion and absorption as well as microbiology and yeast. It is a wonderful test that determines if there is inflammation, digestive issues, and parasitic infection. It also tells us what beneficial and pathogenic bacteria are growing in the intestines.

17. A lot of patients have a need for zinc. The metabolic pathway from norepinephrine to dopamine requires zinc. Mercury is an element like Zinc—a divalent cation. If zinc is insufficient or mercury overabundant, then the pathway will substitute mercury, and the conversion does not happen. Poof! Brain chemical dysfunction. There is often an imbalanced zinc/copper ratio as well. Providing zinc helps keep copper in balance and prevents mercury substitution in a neurochemical process.

18. There are glutamate abnormalities in these patients as well. They tend to spill it in their urine. Some may be missing a necessary rate-limiting enzyme that helps convert glutamine to its metabolites. Others may simply make too much. At any rate, the excess glutamate can cause neurological symptoms.

19. Speech, OT, PT, and behavior therapy are mandatory, as they are a mainstay for improvement.

20. Different combinations of therapies do help. There is a lot that is trial and error and there are a lot of different options. I tell parents to surf the web. If they find something that seems to ring true for their child, then talk to me about it. There is no one right answer for all these patients. While their presentations are rather uniform, their response to therapy is not.

21. I am very clear about what I know and what I do not know. I walk *with* patients, not ahead of them. I am willing to try different therapies as long as there is some information available, if it seems reasonable, and if it will not hurt the child.

22. I will consult with physicians out of state who have treated some of our patients.

Summary

1. Good history and physical.
2. Gluten Free Casein Free Diet. (GFCF)
3. Cod Liver Oil (Rich in vitamin A and Omega three fatty acids)
4. Multivitamin.
5. Probiotics long-term.
6. Vitamin B12: administered transdermally or by injection.
7. Glutathione (potent antioxidant) transdermally.
8. PT/OT/Speech/Behavior therapies
9. Consider chelation of heavy metals with DAN doctors for those really burdened children not responding to gentler methods.
10. Genetics testing (genomics). This can help determine if there are specific genetic problems with methylation, sulfation, and homocysteine metabolism. Looking specifically for the MTHFR gene and glutathione metabolism.

11. Neuroscience testing for neurotransmitter imbalance.
12. Consider homeopathic remedies Carcinosin and Silica.
13. No further vaccines.
14. Measles Mumps Rubella titers.
15. Routine labs: CBC, CMP, thyroid, homocysteine, lipid profile, thyroid testing (free T4 and TSH), urine methylmalonic acid (looking for B12 deficiency.)
16. Brain mapping with professionals trained in neurofeedback.
17. Dried Blood Analysis to pick up fungal overgrowth, heavy metal burden, and digestive issues.
18. Complete Diagnostic Stool Analysis through Genova Diagnostics.
19. Anti-seizure meds if prescribed by a neurologist. Often autistic spectrum patients benefit from anti-epileptic meds even if they do NOT have any evidence of seizures.
20. Spectracell is a blood test that looks at twenty-eight nutrients. It takes three weeks to get the results, as the white cells are grown and then nutrients added or subtracted to see what specific insufficiencies exist at the cellular level.
21. ALCAT (or other) food allergy testing.
22. Consult with a Chinese Medicine specialist can also yield valuable insight and treatment options.

Below are some very helpful websites.
1. www.ICDRC.org—Dr. Jeff Bradstreet
2. www.Wholisticpeds.com—Dr. David Berger (board certified pediatrician)
3. www.drbuttar.com—Dr. Rashid Buttar
4. www.autismresearchinstitute.com
5. www.glycodocs.org

6. www.discovermagazine.com -a great article on how the gut and brain are connected. <u>Autism: It's Not Just in the Head</u>. March 2007

7. www.drneubrander.com Dr. James Neubrander

8. www.learningandachievement.com—Alicia Braccia M.A. C.A.S.

9. www.handle.org

There are many books and resources available on this subject. I have merely scratched the surface to show what can be accomplished in the primary care setting.

Dried Blood Assessment

Dried blood assessment is an alternative method of evaluation that can help provide indications of current health issues and identify potential weaknesses in body systems. The assessment is performed by pricking the finger and collecting drops of blood (ideally eight to ten drops) on a microscope slide. The blood drops are then allowed to dry. Each drop represents one layer of tissue activity in the body, with the first drop representing the current level of health in the body and the successive drops representing deeper layers and exposing potential issues.

Blood is the life force of the body, with a never-ending job of transporting nutrients to and removing waste from each cell of our being, passing through every organ, vessel, muscle, and bone. The information that we can learn from the blood is astounding, and the interpretation and assessment of the findings on the slide are performed by a microscopist specially trained in this field. It is fortunate that we have access to this type of assessment. A report, including microscope pictures of the blood sample, is sent back for every client who submits one for evaluation.

I find this form of assessment very useful, because its primary function is to determine the imbalances present in the body, which we talk about as symptoms. There are four primary root causes behind "why" our bodies' chemistries become unbalanced so that we experience symptoms. They are Candida (yeast overgrowth), parasites, virus, and bacteria. There are other factors to consider as well. Some of these include genetics, emotional stressors, hormonal changes, environmental or chemical toxin exposure, diet, and exercise, to name a few.

To get the most out of this assessment, it is recommended that it be repeated every two to three months, with three assessments being the average needed to identify and address the root issue(s) and stressors causing the body to exhibit the symptoms for which you sought help. This requires a certain amount of patience and persistence, as it takes some time for the body to heal. The general equation to follow is three months to address the issue plus one month for every year the condition has existed for tissue repair. The therapies recommended generally include, but are not limited to herbal preparations, probiotics, colloidal minerals, homeopathic remedies, Bach Flower remedies, detoxification baths, and other non-medication therapies to nourish the body so it can heal.

I, personally, am not trained in doing the interpretation of dried blood samples, but I can share some of what I've learned from results utilizing dried blood assessment. The blood cells should be a healthy red color and well formed, easy to see as individuals, due to a well-connected fibrin network. Fibrin is a protein with the appearance of a spider web, enabling the cells to separate from each other.

The center of each drop represents the digestive area, which makes sense, since digestion is literally at the center of the body. Digestion and assimilation of nutrients affects every one of our body's processes. Looking out from the center, in concentric circles we can see, skin as the outermost layer; then the lymphatic system, endocrine system, connective tissues, and digestion at the center. That is the basic body system's structure of each drop. There are several detailed indications that can then be observed as well, which are too numerous to go into here. Just like fingerprints, no two blood samples are alike.

Here is a short list of several observations that have come back on dried blood assessments:

1. Blood appearance—consistent form to cells as well as color; vibrant red is best. Brown cells indicate lack of oxygenation.
2. The size of the red cells should be consistent. Tightly formed cells indicate nervous system stress.
3. Fibrin network should be well connected. Immune system stress is suspected otherwise. Fibrin is a filamentous protein (I think of spider web) that separates the red cells from each other.
4. White areas within the blood sample generally indicate inflammation. These are called PPP or polymerized protein puddles and are unusable protein stored in the connective tissue because the body cannot get rid of them.
5. Black areas within the blood sample generally indicate congestion.
6. Black star-like shapes within the blood sample generally indicate liver stress.
7. Dark circular bands (like cellulite) indicate the presence of heavy metals. Specific metals are not able to be identified using this assessment. Metals of any kind impede all the systems and keep them from functioning properly, due to their ability to block neurotransmitters from communicating with each other.
8. Lymphatic congestion is observed just inside the skin ring, and it often contains cells that are swollen and bulbous looking; indicating that either the body's ability to detoxify itself by utilizing the four channels of elimination is compromised OR that something is overloading this system. The four channels of elimination are the skin, kidneys, lungs, and colon.
9. Fungal overgrowth makes the cells indistinct, and gives the blood a cloudy appearance.
10. Intestinal dysfunction shows up as microscopic fat particles in the center of the drop, indicating a

leaky gut and compromised digestion, which leads to lymphatic congestion. Poor transport of nutrients like silicon and magnesium can also be seen on the DBA.

11. Parasitic activity is evident by the observation of their waste, which looks like black pencil points throughout the sample; but is usually observed in the digestive area.
12. Viral activity is observed by seeing black polka dots and lines within the PPPs or white areas.
13. Structural issues can be observed by seeing black lines cutting through the sample or the appearance of the perimeter of the drop being pushed out.
14. The brain area is represented at the top of each drop, which is particularly useful to know when heavy metals are involved.

When the body is compromised or exhibiting symptoms of un-wellness, the dried blood assessment can assist us in looking within the body to see:

1. What the general appearance of the blood is,
2. What body systems may be affected,
3. Any specific indications (such as listed above) that are contributing to the breakdown of function.

This information, along with clinical observations of symptoms exhibited by each client, provides a good basis for the microscopist to confidently follow through with the individualized recommendations made, as well as any other therapies he or she believes would be useful.

As stated earlier, it takes time to heal. Modern medicine has done us a disservice with pills that treat symptoms in many illnesses instead of getting to the root of the issue. The importance of relieving our symptoms so that we can feel better quickly is important in our daily lives, but at what cost to our long-term health? It is my belief that addressing the underlying issues and investing the time and finances needed to restore health are all vital components to restoring internal harmony.

SCFranzMD/Carol Matzos

Heavy Metals

Heavy metal burden or heavy metal toxicity has made it into the general medical language in the last few years. This concept is now a common concern for many patients, especially children with ADD/ADHD, autism, and severe allergies.

Many patients have heavy metal burden that is identified in the dried blood assessment. This is interpreted as a "burden" as none of us should have *detectable* heavy metals in our systems. Heavy metal burden means that there has been a slow accumulation and persistence of heavy metals in the body. This burden can cause subtle problems and interfere with cognitive abilities, the endocrine system, and the immune system. In response to the heavy metals, the body develops a systemic fungal infection to buffer the metals. The fungal overgrowth then creates other health problems.

This is not heavy metal "toxicity." True toxicity implies an acute poisoning, or ongoing access to heavy metal ingestion, with very serious symptoms and the need for acute chelation in the emergency setting. Chelation is the use of strong medication to bind the metals. The chelating agents can cause problems themselves if not used carefully by someone with experience in this area.

Where do these metals come from? In young children, it is most likely that the biggest transfer comes through the placenta in utero. After birth, many people simply lack the ability to eliminate the daily accumulation efficiently. This inability or insufficiency can be an inherent genetic problem or can be an acquired issue. Heavy metals are in our food, such as, tuna, swordfish, mackerel, and kingfish; in our water, in our food, and in the air. Air pollution and car exhaust contribute a lot. There is no evidence based research telling us the exact origins of these heavy metal accumulations.

<u>Which heavy metals are these</u>? The most common heavy metals seen are mercury, lead, cadmium, thallium, uranium, barium, arsenic, antimony, aluminum, tin, and nickel. In reality, it doesn't matter if the metals are specifically identified because supplements bind and eliminate most of the heavy metals (it may be that the supplements eliminate all the metals, but in medicine nothing is 100 percent). Early on, I tried to investigate the origins of these heavy metals and why some people have more than others, and I was unable to find any concrete answers. It is enough to know they are there and more importantly, to have a way to rid the body of them. There are plenty of expensive tests that may identify what kinds of metals these are, but the expense is not worth it when they have to be eliminated anyway. These more expensive tests are not offered through this practice.

<u>How do we get rid of them?</u> It is our experience that the herbs recommended through the Dried Blood Assessment offer a gentle form of chelation. Spirulina, chlorella, and omega three fatty acids all help gently bind and eliminate these heavy metals. If a patient needs more aggressive chelation, we refer them to a doctor with experience in this form of therapy. This practice is not comfortable with the more sophisticated forms of chelation (transdermal, IV, rectal, etc.). Aggressive chelation is best done by DAN (Defeat Autism Now) specialists who have more experience and who do research on the subject as well.

<u>Once we get rid of them, will they return</u>? People with elevated cholesterol who have successfully altered their diet to lower their cholesterol can cause it to go up again if they revert to eating the "bad foods." Heavy metals can re-accumulate if one engages in activities that are known to be risk factors for heavy metal accumulation. Said another way, once eliminated, they should not build up rapidly if you are not engaging in high risk behaviors for heavy metal burden. Eating mercury rich foods, hanging out at smelting plants, jogging in traffic, etc., are examples of risky behaviors that cause heavy metals to build back up. Having a "tune up" once a year, in the form of the Dried Blood Assessment, once the metals are gone will help stay on

top of any re-accumulation. Avoiding the obvious sources will also help.

Remarkable success has been made on the supplements recommended in the Dried Blood Assessments. We hope that your child will also experience success and improved health.

ADHD

Everyone has heard of ADHD these days. There is ADHD, Attention Deficit Hyperactivity Disorder, or ADD, Attention Deficit Disorder. It is not an isolated problem and it almost always has an associated dysfunction along with it. This means that there is usually another issue alongside the ADD/ADHD, like obsessive-compulsive disorder, anxiety, depression, and obstinate defiance, etc.

Because I believe it is truly a neurotransmitter imbalance, it is no surprise that there may be these other associated problems alongside the attention issues.

ADD/ADHD is also not a disease. It is a conglomeration of symptoms that have become a common disorder that can be treated with stimulant medications. The commonly known ADD medicines include Ritalin, Metadate (long-acting Ritalin), Concerta, Adderall, Daytrana (long-acting Ritalin), Strattera, and new Vyvanse. All these medications increase the neurotransmitters Norepinephrine and Dopamine. Strattera is the only one of these medications that is not a stimulant, and it affects only norepinephrine. The stimulants act paradoxically in ADD patients and slow their neurotransmissions rather than speed them up. Therefore, the patient typically experiences more focused attention, less anxiety, and more emotional stability.

Up to one-third of gifted children will have allergies and/or ADD. It is more common in boys than girls, and has a strong genetic component (meaning one of the parents or their first degree relatives—aunts, uncles, grandparents—had it as well). It is my experience that many ADD patients have food allergies and heavy metal burden.

Since patients with neurotransmitter imbalance, ADD, ADHD, or whatever label you desire, have less severe but similar symptoms as the autistic patients, many of the evaluation and treatment suggestions are the same. If you consider that all the neurotransmitter imbalances lie on one line or spectrum, you can then define that those with less severe symptoms are at the high end, and those with worse symptoms are at the lower end. This concept gives rise to the term Autistic Spectrum Disorder. Most autistic patients, as they recover, will experience ADD symptoms. Obviously, not every patient with ADD is autistic, either. The point is simply that patients experience many of the same problems along this spectrum of symptoms.

Most of the parents I see who suspect their children have ADD really do not want their children medicated. Some staggering statistics contribute to this problem. There was an article in one of the major magazines like *Times* or *Newsweek* several years ago that stated 90 percent of the world's Ritalin is used in the United States. (I tried googling it and could not find it. I was so disappointed!) There seems to be a general opinion that ADD is over diagnosed in this country, and maybe it is. However, many children do have symptoms, and these children do need help! I encourage parents not to refuse medications if they are indicated. Medication can provide us with valuable information (especially if they make a positive difference!). Medications are not forever. Sometimes children are in crisis with their symptoms. They might be failing in school or be on the verge of being suspended or expelled for behavioral problems that stem from impulse control issues from the ADD/ADHD. In these situations, medication is a must. It is a "quick fix" and can buy time while we look for the "root cause."

Many bright children can compensate for their ADD for many years. It is common to see children begin to decompensate when school finally becomes harder, and they can no longer hide behind their intelligence. Struggles can begin any time, but it is common to see problems arise in fourth grade, seventh, or tenth grade when the child can no longer hold it together.

Another red flag to me is the student who is called lazy. Many high school children are told they are not living up to their potential, or are lazy. Whenever I hear this, I want to get a more detailed history and consider evaluating for ADD. One of my son's friends was not diagnosed until he was a freshman in college. Adderall changed his life for the better.

With the testing we have available, we can investigate for heavy metal issues, fungal overgrowth, neurotransmitter imbalance, vitamin deficiencies, and digestion issues. We can treat these problems with appropriate supplements and begin the process of cleaning and detoxifying the body.

Most of the therapies, tests, and recommendations in the autism information above are also applied to investigating and treating ADD/ADHD. The most important concept I can convey is that there usually are options available. Having choices can be a very valuable asset, because there is not a magic remedy that fixes everything. It is a process of healing; a journey that is worth taking.

Anorexia Nervosa (AN)/Eating Disorder (ED)

Anorexia Nervosa (AN) has been around a long time. It was poorly understood in the past, but has become more common and is a devastating disorder both physically and mentally. In my early years of practice, I never saw it. In the last ten years, I have had many cases, with the youngest being ten and the oldest seventeen. Two patients have been males, and the worst case was a fourteen-year-old female. Karen Carpenter is one of the more famous people with AN. In the movie *White Christmas* with Bing Crosby, Rosemary Clooney, and Vera Ellen, Vera had AN. Her neck skin was so flabby from weight loss that all her outfits had turtlenecks to hide it. No one knew what was wrong then.

Eating disorders are really difficult to treat and involve a *lot* of emotional therapy. It is all about control! One in four college females are reported to have an eating disorder. AN/ED creates a lot of really ugly behaviors.

What sets it off? That part is poorly understood. In the patients I have treated, all were high achievers who took to heart an offhand comment about weight. Sometimes parents can be inadvertently and negatively focused on weight and create the mindset in their daughter by making her believe she is fat.

Once the eating disorder becomes entrenched, these patients, who are primarily female, become extremely deceitful. They have learned to manipulate every situation and everyone in their lives to protect the eating disorder mindset. This is the only thing they can control, so they believe. It is difficult to believe ANYTHING they tell you. When they come into the office to be seen, I require they be in shorts and a T-shirt. Anorexic patients will load up with water before they come in just to increase their weight. They will put weights on their ankles if in long pants. Their eyes are dark, empty, and they are obsessed with not being fat. I had one girl tell me she would rather die than be fat. Patients begin to restrict how much they eat. They will want to eat alone in their rooms and not with the family or groups of friends. They count calories, fear fats in foods, and offset any calorie intake with intense and prolonged exercise.

It is important to enlist the help of a nutritionist and counselor with experience in the field of eating disorders. Eating disorders are all about control, and usually the inciting event is some insignificant comment someone made about being overweight. Someone said something about being too heavy and, bam, the patient took it to heart and began restricting her food intake. Even as the physician, I have been deceived and manipulated, and I learned from it. I learned that the medical person involved becomes the last bastion for these patients when outpatient therapy does not help. When a patient returns to me from the nutritionist, it is because she is failing and needs to have an NG (nasogastric) feeding tube placed to ensure adequate calorie intake. The patient may have to wear the NG tube to school and may even feel humiliated. Unfortunately at this juncture, I am not sympathetic to the plight because it is about saving the patient's life. Usually at that point, she needs inpatient therapy in a facility experienced in the treatment of eating disorders.

The BEST inpatient facility in the nation, at this time, is Remuda with facilities in Virginia and Arizona. It is expensive, but this is a bad disease and not just anyone can treat it.

Many of the community hospitals are ill equipped to deal with an eating disorder, as it is primarily psychiatric in nature. The psychiatric facilities are not very experienced in eating disorders. ED (eating disorder) patients *cannot* be treated the same as other patients with other psychiatric illnesses. When a patient needs admission to the community hospital, it is for medical management. This includes electrolyte management and stabilization of medical issues stemming from the eating disorder. Once stabilized, the patient needs inpatient therapy in a facility that deals with this issue.

I do not treat this illness homeopathically.

Cardiovascular complications are common in patients with anorexia nervosa, occurring in up to 80 percent of patients. Bradycardia (slow heart rate), low blood pressure (hypotension), arrhythmias, repolarization abnormalities, and sudden death are among these complications. QT abnormalities (an EKG heart rhythm problem) may also occur as well as changes in myocardial mass and function. (Olivares JL, *Eur Journal Pediatrics*, published online 03/15/05.)

Treating eating disorders is labor intensive, emotionally draining, and time consuming. It usually takes all our resources to care for these patients properly. It may require Baker acting (involuntarily admitting a patient to the hospital) a patient to get the therapeutic ball rolling. These patients are usually hateful, belligerent, defiant, and negative.

In summary:

1. This is a bad disorder.
2. The patient cannot be trusted to tell you the truth once the eating disorder is well established. It is important that the healthcare providers and the family not be caught in the web of lies the patient will weave.
3. When visiting the medical office, the patient needs to be weighed in wearing as little clothing as possible at every visit. Shorts and a T-shirt are fine. This way

there can be no hidden weights to falsely increase the weight to keep the provider from seeing weight loss.

4. Newly diagnosed patients need immediate consultation with a nutritionist and a therapist with experience in eating disorders. If the patient does not respond to nutritional intervention, then she may need an NG (nasogastric tube) placed. It can be done as on outpatient. If the patient has reached a point of collapse, developed bradycardia (low heart rate), or has lost greater than or equal to 10 percent of their body weight, then she needs to be admitted for medical management until inpatient placement can be done.

5. Placement is expensive (around $40,000 and up), and Remuda is our first choice. Often insurance pays little, or not enough. However, without proper treatment, one in seven girls will die from this illness.

6. We are not the patient's "friend." We are here to provide aggressive medical management despite her protests. Aggressive measures, including Baker Acting a patient or involving the Department of Children and Families, might be needed if the patient's life is endangered.

7. The patient will whine, wheedle, manipulate, and make promises she does not keep. I learned that the hard way. Treatment is not negotiable.

8. Eating disorder patients lose bone density and develop amenorrhea (periods stop). Menses is the last thing to correct even after weight has stabilized; it may take up to two years for the hormones to straighten out, and for menses to resume normally.

9. Women die from this condition if it is untreated. Once identified, therapy needs to be swift and aggressive for the best outcome. This problem sneaks up on families. What I have outlined is harsh reality.

I hope that it helps parents, friends, and family to be more aware and tuned into their children's eating habits and attitudes. If there are *any* concerns at all, get your child evaluated. It is better to be wrong than to be right and let the disorder become entrenched.

10. The good news is that more people are aware of this issue and there are more resources available so that recovery is more likely to happen.

Chapter Seven

Getting Started With Chinese Medicine

Chinese medicine has been around for approximately 5,000 years. Anything with such a long track record has to have some validity! Acupuncture and Chinese medicine view the body differently than western medicine does. Chinese medicine is based on body systems, and it divides them into mind, body, and soul. Many aspects of this medicine can be described and treated only in the living person, as many signs of illness are not found after death.

Western medicine is based more on anatomy, chemistry, and physiology, and has a tendency to compartmentalize the body rather than view it as a whole. Much of western medicine pathology has been described from the anatomy after death.

Chinese medicine works off energy meridians and organ dysfunction. The internal organs and nature of the body are also connected to the outside environment, and the internal affects the external, and vice versa.

When an organ experiences changes during illness, the organ that corresponds to a sick organ will go through similar changes. Chinese medicine practitioners observed these changes and created a system that uses wood, fire, earth, metal, and water as symbols to describe the body system.

In Chinese medicine, the internal organs are divided into hollow organs—stomach, gallbladder, small intestine, large intestine, and bladder; and solid organs—heart, lungs, liver, spleen, and kidneys. Each organ is also attached to an earth element—earth, fire, water, metal, and wood. The brain is not an organ in Chinese medicine as it is considered the consciousness of the person.

The pairings are as follow:

Stomach / spleen / earth
Kidney / bladder / water
Heart / small intestine / fire
Liver / gallbladder /wood
Lungs/ large intestine / metal.

1. Wood represents the beginning of growth. It is represented by the color green and the season spring. The liver and gallbladder are related to wood. Liver detoxifies the blood and stores blood in Chinese medicine. In the winter, more blood is required to keep the internal organs warm, and in the summer, less is required. The extra returns to the liver and the excess energy is used to repair the body. Wood also represents anger. The liver is considered the seat of all emotion and people with low liver energy are easily angered. The term bilious derives from this association.

2. Fire represents flourishing and growth. It is associated with the color red. So is the heart. The season is summer when plant growth is at its peak. The heart and small intestine are associated with this element of nature. It is associated with heat. In the summer, heat needs to be dissipated. When the heat is too high in the summer, the heart is at risk for injury. As above, the excess energy from the blood is used for repair in the summer. The heart is repaired during the early

morning hours. Illnesses that affect the heart will also affect the small intestine.

3. Earth is associated with a damp and humid environment. The spleen and stomach are the organs paired with this element. The season is end of summer. The color is yellow. Worry is associated with these organs and this element. Overly anxious people can have a damaged spleen, and a damaged spleen leads to anxiety. Many stomach ailments occur at the end of summer. In Chinese medicine, this is the body repairing the stomach. In western medicine, it marks the beginning of school and shared viruses.

4. Metal represents depression and melancholy; being solemn and sad or sorrowful emotionally. The season is autumn. The color is white. The organs are lung and large intestine. A person with weak lungs is sorrowful. Autumn is associated with respiratory illness. This is true as every fall, between October and the end of November, we see a ton of respiratory problems. Asthma, allergies, and influenza often rule in the fall. Allergy-Immune-Respiratory Tea A.I.R. Tea) is an incredible asset during this time.

5. Water represents coldness. The season associated with it is winter. The organs are the kidneys and bladder. The color is black. The kidneys are the only solid organs not protected by the rib cage. They require the most blood flow in the winter to keep warm. Kidneys are said to be the organs of life. They carry the energy of life in Chinese medicine. The emotion associated with it is FEAR.

Chinese Medicine also sees that foods and medicines have characteristics associated with them that can help us treat patients. Foods and medicines are hot, warm, neutral, cool, or cold natured. When a patient is hot natured then cold natured foods and medicines are indicated. If a patient is cold then they need hot. Very common sense. By seeing a trained Chinese medicine physician, you can begin to alter your diet, medications, and begin the return to balanced and harmonious health.

Well, that is all I know about Chinese medicine. It is enough to make you think and to see how our bodies are connected to our external world. It is interesting because when we see our bodies as more than the sum of its parts, we can see connections that influence us. This enables us to make better health choices and to understand the consequences or results of such choices.

For example, western medications are generally warm to hot. They produce heat in the body. In a sensitive person with liver energy, too much heat of the wood will cause internal fire or a fever (like rubbing sticks together with flint). Some medications can cause drug fever in certain patients. This gives a little insight into the possible reasons of medication side effects. Yeast rashes from antibiotics happen because the medicine was hot natured and dried up body fluids, which led to a rash.

Coumadin thins the blood. What makes viscous fluid thin? Heat. Therefore, coumadin is a hot natured medicine. Very interesting, is it not?

Below are four Chinese herbal products that produce amazing results on the body. The ingredients and actions are listed. You can see the traditional Chinese medicine affects as well the western medicine interpretation of the same.

Si Jin Bao, Inc.
Four Golden Treasures, Inc.

Mei Mao (Wonderful)

Ingredients
Distilled Water, Witch Hazel, Apricot Kernel Oil, Sweet Almond
Oil, Bees Wax, Vegetable Glycerin, Shan Yao (Chinese Yam),
Xia Ku Cao (Prunella Spike), Bei Zi Cao (Lithospermum Root),
Sha Shen (Glehnia Root), Shi Chang Pu (Acorus Rhizome) Ru
Xiang(Frankincense), Wu Wei Zi (Schisandra Fruit), Bing Pian
(Menthol), Alcohol (Plant Source)

Actions:

TCM	Western
Firms the Skin	Restores Elasticity: Improves Collagen
Reduces inflammation	Skin Hydrator
Promotes regeneration	Anti-Oxidizing
Tonifies Qi	Anti-Aging
Clears Heat	Improves Microcirculation
Promotes regeneration of the Flesh	Restores Youthful Appearance
Tones the Musculature	Makes skin supple

Indications
- Lessen fine lines and wrinkles
- Firm & tone skin
- Reduce cellulite

Commentary:

Wonderful is an herbal cream used to tone and firm the skin. Patients are always asking for ways to look younger and this formula was created specifically to do that. Wonderful will tone and firm the skin anywhere on the body and reduce cellulite. It is also especially effective at removing wrinkles. Unlike Botox or other topical treatments, after ninety days, Wonderful's effects will last even without further treatment. Continued use will maintain and enhance results. We find this is especially popular with our Acupuncture Facelift patients.

Course of Treatment

For best results, use 1.5cc-2.0cc on or near affected area once daily.

www.SJBHERBS.com   407-682-HERB Fax 407-574-6834

Si Jin Bao, Inc.
Four Golden Treasures, Inc.

Fu Xing (Revive)

Ingredients

Distilled Water, Alcohol (Plant Source), Apricot Kernel Oil, Sweet Almond Oil, Bees Wax, Vegetable Glycerin, Lecithin, Bai Ji Tian (Morinda Root), Bing Pian (Menthol), Chang Pu (Acorus Rhizome), Chi Shao (Red Peony Root), Chuan Xiong (Ligustricum), Du Zhong (Eucommia Bark), Fang Feng (Siler Root), Huang Qi (Astralagus Root), Mo Yao (Myrrh), Ru Xiang(Mastic Frankincense), Sheng Di(Raw Rehmannia Root), Wei Ling Xian (Clematis), Wu Wei Zi (Schisandra Fruit), Xu Duan (Marsh Plant)

Actions:

TCM	Western
Invigorate Qi	Increases Micro-Circulation
Eliminate Cold	Increases Lymphatic Circulation
Move Blood Flow	Increases Capillary Circulation
Eliminate Bi	Promote regeneration of the flesh
Open the collaterals	Anti -Inflammatory
Relax the Sinews	Analgesic
Reduces Swelling	

Indications

• Baggy Eyes	• Prelude to Wonderful Treatment**
• Lost of Luster	• Joint Sprains
• Pale Complexion	• Muscle Strains
• Bumps	• Headache

• Pain of any type	• Joint Sprains
• Acute or Chronic	• Bumps
• Bruises	• Joint Pain

Commentary:

Alleviates pain of any type. Originally designed as a preventative measure for the muscle strain caused by performing too many Tuina (Chinese massage) sessions. We also found it to be great for our clients as well. It quickly works to invigorate the microcirculation.

Course of Treatment

For best results, use 1.5cc-2.0cc on or near affected area three times daily for ninety days

www.SJBHERBS.com   407-682-HERB Fax 407-574-6834

Si Jin Bao, Inc.
Four Golden Treasures, Inc

Guang Hua (Schmoove)

Ingredients

Distilled Water, Witch Hazel, Apricot Kernel Oil, Sweet Almond Oil, Bees Wax, Vegetable Glycerin, Da Huang (Rhubarb Root), Di Fu Zi (Kocia Fruit), Bei Zi Cao (Lithospermum Root), Cang Er Zi (Xanthium Fruit), Huang Qin (Scutellaria (Skullcap) Root), Hong Hua (Safflower), Chi Shao Yao (Red Peony Root – Cooked), Huang Qi (Astralagus Root), Sha Shen (Glehnia Root), Bo He (Peppermint Oil), Alcohol(Plant Source)

Actions:

TCM	Western
Disperses Summer Heat	Regenerates the flesh
Eliminates Wind	Dries Oily Skin
Dries Dampness	Promote Microcirculation
Nourish Yin fluid	Enhances Cell Repair
Clears Heat	Promotes Healthy Skin Growth
Clears Damp Heat	Reduces Inflammation
Promote Qi Circulation	Helps Skin return moisture and produce natural Oils

Indications

- Dry skin
- Dermatitis
- Eczema
- Athlete's Foot
- Age spots
- Rosacea
- Sunburn

Commentary:

This herbal cream treats many types of skin conditions. Clinically it has been successful in treating many types of dermatitis, which include acne, eczema, rosacea, sunburns, scrapes, bug bites, and more. It should be used three times a day for optimal results. Only a small amount is needed, and it can be used as a close as 20 minutes apart between doses.

www.SJBHERBS.com   407-682-HERB   Fax 407-574-6834

Si Jin Bao, Inc.
Four Golden Treasures, Inc

Zhi Suo Bu Zheng Qi Tang
Formerly (Zhi Sou Bu Pi Fei Shen Tang)

Stop Cough & Immuno-Support Tea
(Renamed A.I.R. for Allergy-Immune-Respiratory Tea)

Ingredients
Distilled Water, Sheng Jiang (Fresh Ginger), Jie Geng (Platycodon), Che Qian Qian Zi (Plantago Seed), Hou Po (Magnolia Bark), Bu Gu Zhi (Psoralea Fruit), Bei Sha Shen (Glehnia Root), Cang Er Zi (Xanthium Fruit), Bai Zhi (Dahurien Angelica), Xin Yi Hua (Magnolia Flower), Glycerin (Plant Source)

Actions:

<u>TCM</u>	<u>Western</u>
Allow Lungs to grasp Qi	Anti-histamine
Nourishes production of Yin & Yang	Anti-spasmodic
Resolve Phlegm	Anti-emetic
Transform Phlegm	Anti-inflammatory
Eliminate Phlegm	Functions like Anti-biotic
Open the Nose	Functions like Anti-viral
Rectifies the Qi	Stomachic
	Expectorant

Indications
- All types of Asthma
- All types Cough
- Rhinitis
- Sinusitis (including sinus infection)

- Seasonal Allergies (itchy, watery eyes, itchy nose, etc.)
- Certain types of Uticaria (Differential Diagnosis Required)

Commentary:

This formula is designed to eliminate any upper-respiratory and/or sinus conditions. The formula was originally designed several years ago at the request of a local holistic pediatrician who was looking for something to stop coughs and clear infections that also tasted good.

www.SJBHERBS.com   407-682-HERB   Fax 407-574-6834

Made in the USA
Columbia, SC
22 March 2018